Dental Care for the Elderly

Dental Care for the Elderly

Editors

Bertram Cohen
DDS, FDS, FRC Path.

and

Hamish Thomson
HDD, FDS

YEAR BOOK MEDICAL PUBLISHERS, INC.
Chicago · London · Boca Raton

First published in 1986 by
William Heinemann Medical Books Ltd,
22 Bedford Square, London WC1B 3HH
© 1986 Bertram Cohen and Hamish Thomson

Library of Congress Cataloging-in-Publication Data

Dental care for the elderly.

Includes bibliographies and index.
1. Aged—Dental care.   I. Cohen, Bertram.
II. Thomson, Hamish. [DNLM: 1. Dental Care—in
old age.   2. Geriatric Dentistry. WU 490 D4141]
RK55.A3D46 1987   617.6′00880565   87–6295
ISBN 0–8151–1815–5

Typeset by D. P. Media Hitchin
Printed in Great Britain by
Redwood Burn Limited,
Trowbridge, Wiltshire

Contents

List of Contributors

H. M. Bramley MA, BM, ChB
Greenhills,
Back Lane,
Hathersage
Sheffield

W. H. Binnie DDS, MSD, FDS, MRC Path.
Professor and Chairman
Department of Pathology
Baylor College of Dentistry
3302 Gaston Ave
Dallas, Texas 75246

B. Cohen DDS, FDS, FRC Path., Hon FRCS
Royal College of Surgeons
35–43 Lincoln's Inn Fields, London

M. R. P. Hall MA, BM, BCh, FRCP
Professor of Geriatric Medicine
Centre Block (Level E)
Southampton General Hospital

R. J. Ibbetson BDS, MSc, FDS
Eastman Dental Hospital
Gray's Inn Road, London

R. B. Johns PhD, LDS
Charles Clifford Dental School
University of Sheffield

Hamish Thomson HDD, FDS
57 Portland Place, London

J. M. Wright, DDS, MS
Associate Professor of Pathology
Baylor College of Dentistry

Preface

No spring nor summer beauty hath such grace
As I have seen in one autumnal face.

John Donne

This book has its origins in a meeting held at the Royal College of Surgeons of England in 1983. An all day symposium entitled 'Three Score Years and Then?' was devoted to Dentistry's last priority and, despite the gloomy forebodings of those who predicted that there would be no audience for a topic of this sort, the attendance exceeded the previous highest for meetings in this series. We interpreted this response as recognition of the growing need for devoting more time and more attention to elderly patients. Hitherto the teaching of dentistry and of dental public health education has directed an overwhelming preponderance of its attention to childhood and early adolescence, to the extent that care for the elderly has come to be neglected – both relatively and absolutely.

The current increase in numbers of the elderly has resulted from improved social conditions, advances in the control of illnesses formerly fatal and more positive medical care. Death is no longer taken for granted after 70 and a greater effort is made by sons and daughters, often in their fifties and sixties, to provide room and board, comfort and compassion for their parents and more of this will be required in the years to come when many of today's middle-aged population, spared from wars and epidemics, reach the often youthful age of 70 with the prospect of 20 years ahead.

According to the 1981 census, 17.7% of the British population were of pensionable age. Of these the highest proportion was in the Southwest (20.7%) and the lowest in the West Midlands (16.1%). The expectation of life at birth has risen to 76 years for women and 70 for men. The number of those over 75 is expected to continue rising up to 1986 when women will outnumber men in a ratio of 3:1. The greatest percentage increase will be in those of 85 and over (43.5%). The absolute numbers of those over 75 will rise from 2 280 000 to 3 000 000 by 1991 and the over 85s will increase from 400 000 to 600 000 by the year 2000.

The young elderly (between 65 and 74) do not differ markedly in health status from the younger population, but after 75 disease and death rates rise steeply. One-fifth of those aged 85 and over are housebound or permanently in bed and mental infirmity in this group presents a serious problem; 2% have severe visual impairment and 3% have difficulty with hearing. Women have a greater expectation of life and two-thirds of women over the age of 75 are widows. Undue concentrations of lonely and isolated old people exist in the inner zones of large cities and in retirement areas. To assume that they are invariably members of a family group is a mistake that can lead to their being overlooked despite the best intentions to care for them.

It is disturbing to read in medical literature of the high proportion of elderly patients suffering from dental disability. Advice on care of the teeth often has to be provided by the medical practitioner, as part of total medical care. Neglect of oral hygiene and a high proportion of edentulous patients are commonly seen and it is often difficult for geriatricians to find dental practitioners to care for these patients.

Thus challenged, dentists must be encouraged to make their professional skills available to these people. However, it is not enough to be prepared for an occasional domiciliary visit carrying a bag packed with every tool from forceps to facebow. It is necessary to participate in the organisation of dental care not only for the affluent elderly but also for the indigent who are confined to house or institution, so that their appetites may be restored and their appearance blossom again. Such a spark has appeared in several communities, but occasional efforts are not enough and a sustained development is required.

The seven chapters of this book fall into two parts. In the first four chapters an attempt is made to introduce the reader to matters inherently related to ageing – from those affecting the psyche to those that concern the teeth specifically, the soft tissues of the mouth and, finally, to those considerations of nutrition and metabolism without a knowledge of which any attempts at treatment or management are likely to be empirical. Following these theoretical observations, the second half of the book is devoted to treatment of the patient, of his teeth and of the edentulous state. We hope that any repetition of the need for respect and concern will be condoned, for this recurrent theme is indeed the most important single message that our authors have to offer; we recognise, but reject, the view that compassion consumes time and that in present circumstances it has to be regarded as a luxury. It is, in fact, a genuine need.

One of the difficulties in dealing with elderly patients is that they may be frustrated by a lack of ability to describe what is wrong. The dentist has, therefore, to be skilled in transposing what the patient describes into a diagnosis. He must also be alert to the possibility that his patient may shrink from articulating unspoken fears so that an apparently unsubstantiated complaint about a denture could conceal anxiety about the tissues on which it rests.

There are omissions from the text but reasons for them. The tissues of the periodontium are discussed, but the prevention and treatment of periodontal diseases should be undertaken in middle age and earlier. Periodontal lesions are likely to have deteriorated too far for anything more than minor local palliative treatment in the seventies and eighties. The teeth may even have stabilised and will respond to measures such as simple mouthwashes and gingival packs for occasional pain or swelling. It is never too late for hygiene by tape, woodstick or cotton bandage, nor would it be wrong to perform minor occlusal adjustments to prevent the drift of a migrating tooth. The message must be to treat the periodontia of affected teeth in the forties and before with a view to preparing them to survive until old age.

Maxillofacial surgery and associated prostheses are not considered because they belong properly in a more specialised text. Likewise the treatment and after-care required for malignant disease is outside the province of this book, although it has to be emphasised that the dental practitioner has a crucial responsibility for the early recognition of these life-threatening conditions.

The diagnosis and treatment of systemic emergencies and those that may occur during dental operations are omitted because they are well described in such publications as 'Emergencies in Dental Practice' prepared by the Department of Health. This should be read and be to hand in every dental practice, department and domiciliary kit. In it there are appendices on drugs that may precipitate emergencies and on criteria for safety in dental anaesthesia, which receives only passing mention in our text.

It goes without saying that cooperation with the elderly patient's physician is essential and it is the dentist's responsibility to renew and maintain this contact. Finally, it is worth emphasising that short-term attitudes and treatment plans should be avoided for all elderly patients and not merely those who are reluctant to accept the prospect of old age. They need all the encouragement they can receive in order to make the best of their remaining years. The dentist is faced with frequent complaints from elderly patients, many of them seemingly unjustified, but argument and anger are futile. Criticism must be absorbed and every effort made to help. Somehow these elderly nuisances must become old dears.

BC
HT

Acknowledgements

Figures 2.1 and 2.3 are photographs by Mr George Elia, of specimens in the Odontological Museum of the Royal College of Surgeons of England, published by courtesy of the Honorary Curator, Professor A. E. W. Miles. We should also like to thank James Morgan for providing the illustrations in Chapter 7.

The Editors are indebted to Susan Chandler for her considerable and always cheerful help in preparing typescript, checking references, and conducting correspondence with our contributors, and to Miss M. A. Clennett, librarian of the British Dental Association, for her considerable assistance.

Finally, we owe our thanks to Dr Richard Barling of William Heinemann Medical Books for his interest and advice and to Miss Caroline Creed for her help in the later stages of production.

Section I

Chapter 1

Understanding Older Patients

H. M. BRAMLEY

INTRODUCTION

The mention of elderly patients may bring to mind a classic stereotype: unsteady, stiff, slow, not seeing or hearing too well, muddled, fearful, having difficulty in remembering instructions and, what's more, about to cause an irredeemable delay in the day's appointments.

The physiological processes of ageing and the gradual diminution in acuity of the five senses are facts, but the rate at which they occur shows great variation. Some people assume the life of a cabbage and sink into presenile dementia in their fifties, while others maintain the creativity of a Verdi or a Churchill to the end of a long life. Nearer to our time and subject, Winifred Rushforth, in her 97th year, produced a new and significant work on the effect of the unconscious in everyday life.

Unique personality traits tend to become accentuated with age rather than diminished, and the occurrence of marked variations in physical capacity between persons and between bodily systems in the same person make sweeping statements about the elderly and our relationship with them quite untenable. There are only three generalisations worth making: we are born, we die, and in the intervening period we are all different.

Who are the elderly? Perhaps they are persons ten to fifteen years older than the dentist himself. Much of what will be said about understanding older patients applies to any age, but perhaps with the elderly even greater sensitivity is required.

The subject will not be presented in terms of formal psychology, but by illustrations from everyday practice. To aid discussion, the following three headings will be used: attitude of the dentist; the needs and features of older patients; and face-to-face.

THE ATTITUDE OF THE DENTIST

The establishment of helpful relationships between a dentist and his patient is a double-sided process. He must seek not only to understand the patient but to be aware of his own temperament, and also to understand his own feelings, memories and prejudices as they are evoked by the clinical encounter.

Prejudices and anxieties

A difficult old person may remind the dentist of a cantankerous parent who has caused him much trouble and anxiety. The bad feelings so raised may interfere with his treatment.

A patient smelling of alcohol may sit down in the chair, arousing great anxieties in the dentist who has had to suffer an alcoholic spouse or parent. He feels his hackles rise, instead of wanting to understand his patient's difficulties.

Some professional men and women become excessively anxious when criticised. The older patient who says, 'Your treatment has made me worse; I can hardly eat at all now,' may be arousing feelings that the dentist had as a child, being continually criticised by perfectionist parents. Unless hostile feelings are recognised, thought about and understood, the dentist will act on them and emit hostile feelings to the patient. No good work can then be done between them.

Unacknowledged racial prejudice in the clinician, particularly if this is combined with language difficulties experienced by the elderly immigrant, is a recipe for uncaring management.

An overt homosexual can arouse fear or disgust in a dentist who has never really faced up to his own attitudes to homosexuality.

Male and female patients, even when old, can exert their sexuality and can take away professional confidence if the dentist is not quickly aware of what is happening.

> An attractive woman of 63 years of age, in accepting a compliment on her appearance from her much younger dentist, started to tell him in some detail how her husband was always chasing her and how she managed to keep him off except for once a week. The dentist was just about to adjust the chair to a reclining position and put his arm round her head for a dental examination. He was thrown off his professional stance by this confiding and seductive woman.

> A well-preserved elderly man looked into the eyes of his lady dentist and said, 'Do you believe in morals?' Such a remark must be accepted calmly, put in its place and a professional relationship restored, if effective work is to be accomplished.

From time to time, most dentists treat patients suffering from terminal illness. They may be giving the considerable service of achieving mouth comfort or perhaps, as oral surgeons, being concerned with more specialised issues. Some thought should be given to attitudes to death and the dying. Professional people are notoriously bad at facing up to this, and patients and their families often suffer in the web of dishonesty and deception which ultimately springs from the doctor's ignorance of his own emotional preoccupations. Tears, sadness, despair and the inability to cope with 'failure' all encourage him to avoid the truth. He should understand why he is particularly vulnerable and come to terms with the origins within himself, so that he can be straightforwardly supportive to such patients without deceit or anxiety.

Temperament

It is unlikely that any of us has an ideal temperament for dealing with each and every elderly patient. We can, however, be aware of our temperament and know that briskness and ultra-efficiency may be confusing and that gentle, warm optimism is to be preferred to glum frigidity; that physical closeness – the handshake, the hand on the shoulder – is to be preferred to polite formality and distance.

Cheerfulness is to be preferred to the jokiness which can be misinterpreted even though expressed with the best of motives, namely, to relieve tension.

> 'I'm sure I don't know what we're going to do with this odd mouth full of teeth.' The result of this light-hearted remark was that the patient, a retired Inspector of Education, became very anxious that something was seriously wrong and didn't like to ask the dentist. This worried her so much that a few years later she recorded this as one of the worst days in her life!

Each of us is stuck with our own particular temperament, but we should recognise and seek to modify the inappropriate impact of this temperament on elderly patients.

Attitudes to time

Time is money. Are we willing to bear the financial burden of unhurried consultation? Can we make the patient feel we are relaxed enough to listen to and fully understand his difficulties?

Can we regard one of our skills as listening and thinking about the total material the patient presents to us and produce a treatment plan which is entirely appropriate to that individual?

A young dentist being interviewed about the job he was doing with geriatric patients said that he was very dissatisfied. He had been highly trained to do a skilled job and didn't feel he should waste valuable time listening to old people's endless complaints!

If dentistry does not take place in the context of a good, caring relationship, the amount accomplished will actually be less and it is certain that the patient will not be satisfied.

Personal security and avoidance of 'problem-solving' platitudes

Can the dentist be secure enough to be puzzled by a situation, to accept it and not to try to get by with remarks such as, 'Never mind, Mrs Smith; there's no need to worry; we'll soon have this sorted out'? This sometimes reassures the dentist but can make the patient feel that it is unacceptable to mention his real anxieties. It may be that the problem is insoluble and the dentist's most constructive approach is to share and bear the pain with the patient, who is thus given courage to face his problems and carry on. It is not easy to share pain, uncertainty and difficult problems with a patient, and the temptation to come to some unreal or untrue solution must be resisted. This is particularly so with pain and paraesthesia in the distribution of the trigeminal nerve, and with other more bizarre intraoral symptoms that resist all attempts, even at an advanced level, to make a diagnosis.

The dentist may well feel driven to resort to active treatment, which can lead to iatrogenic effects and ever more desperate measures, often with a resulting cascade of disaster.

Coming to terms with his own ageing process

The practising dentist's capacity for sustained and complex clinical work diminishes with age. If this is not recognised, standards will fall. To some extent this can be overcome by careful appointment scheduling, placing the more demanding work at the time of day when he is at his best and allowing ample time for its completion.

The dentist must be aware that a diminution of physical

capacity can subtly influence the quality of treatment planning. Age and experience often bring a more conservative attitude to surgical or dental treatment, and the complex and the ambitious may be set aside in favour of the basic and simple. This 'mature' judgement may, however, be a rationalisation of fading powers and not necessarily in the best interests of the patient.

The older dentist often has useful insights into the management of his elderly patients, but sometimes he will project on to these patients the very things from which he himself suffers, such as increasing indecision, deafness and forgetfulness, without acknowledging that he shares these deficiencies.

A widow, aged 72, made elaborate arrangements with her daughter to be taken to the dentist for 9.15 a.m. only to be told that her appointment was at 2.15 p.m. although the morning appointment had been written in her diary. This was the dentist's mistake but, rather than admit it, he told her she must have heard wrongly. This was not the first mistake he had made with appointments. Instead of acknowledging his own forgetfulness and partial deafness and leaving all the appointment-making to his receptionist, he continued to make such mistakes.

NEEDS AND FEATURES OF OLDER PATIENTS

Rigid attitudes and painful memories

The patient's ideas of dentistry may have been inculcated in youth and never revised. Extractions and dentures may be his idea of the only functions of the dentist. His first contact with a dentist may have been painful, and it may be very difficult to persuade him that dental procedures need not be painful. His ideas and visions of any dental procedure may be completely different from those of the dentist and from reality. The dentist will never know this unless he listens. Reassurance is useless unless the patient's attitudes and fears are understood and he is confident that the dentist has understood them.

The fact that dental care may have benefits for health and happiness may not be appreciated until much unhurried time has been spent with the patient. Defences against fear and pain and the changing of long-held attitudes tend to grow stronger with age.

'Too late to bother'

The mouth is often a mirror in old age of how much care a person is still able to take with the totality of his health and appearance. Chronic disease can lead to neglect of the mouth because of depression and lack of energy. Instructions to the patient must take this into account, and perhaps use can also be made of ancillary help. If the patient is really too tired to comply with instructions, the dentist may have to set his sights lower. On the other hand, some lethargic patients are encouraged by knowing that someone is taking a real interest in them and respond very well to praise, especially if visits are fairly frequent.

Under- and over-reporting of symptoms

There is a certain expectation of discomfort and disability with advancing age, which may result in the under-reporting of symptoms. This can lead to late diagnosis in carcinoma of the mouth. All symptoms, even if they are played down, must be seriously investigated.

Much more frequently, some lonely and miserable old people present with firmly-held complaints, often of the most bizarre symptoms: 'I get a terrible pain down my left leg every time I put in my top teeth'; 'My upper lip burns and burns all the time and it's driving me mad'; 'I get this foul tasting sticky stuff and it comes off in white lumps inside my mouth'; 'The pain throbs and burns and shoots like an electric shock all over my mouth; it is there all the time.' Each of these complaints could come from someone looking physically well and getting eight hours' sleep every night.

Such complaints are fully investigated with (predictably) no physical diagnosis but with the increasing realisation that to be over 80 years of age is a tremendous challenge to which few can rise.

For many people at this age there is increasing isolation, loss of financial independence, family friction, failing physical powers, and the prospect of nothing. It is no wonder that attention and sympathy is claimed subconsciously and that a regular visit to a sympathetic dentist or doctor is part of a 'game' which keeps the individual going.

At this age it is unlikely that psychotherapy will be useful, and a pharmacological approach to a social and human problem may have only peripheral ameliorative effects. The dentist's only helpful role may well be just that of giving time and attentive listening. We certainly make the situation worse by giving unnecessary treatment to salve our own consciences for not being able to help the patient face his deeper problems. Action is a poor substitute for thought in dealing with patients who over-report and make demands for things to be done. Action may be the dentist's defence against failing to understand the patient's needs.

Loss of teeth and other losses

Elderly people may become greatly depressed by their losses – loss of relatives and friends by death, loss of earning capacity, loss of status, loss of possessions on moving to smaller accommodation, and loss of independence. Against this background the prospect of the loss of remaining teeth may have far more horror for them than we can appreciate, being symbolic of the loss of yet another part of themselves. The dentist should listen for the real fears and causes of depression and must help the patient to come to terms with this latest loss. A positive approach may help some patients (e.g. 'You will look so much better, really look younger, and you'll certainly enjoy eating more'). However, this could be regarded by the patient as a facile misunderstanding of the significance to him of tooth loss. In the matter of final extractions, the dentist may be treading on broken glass.

> Mrs M, a formidable lady in her late sixties, has had intense intractable pain in the region of the lower right mental nerve distribution which has filled her whole life since final dental extractions in her mid-fifties. She has had the gamut of consultation and methods of pain relief with no diagnosis and no resolution. It appears that a dental surgery assistant known to her socially had suggested she ought to lose her remaining teeth. The dentist carried this out without fully involving her in the decision. Apart from some slight difficulty with the lower right canine tooth, there were no problems. Shortly afterwards, the pain started and she has never been able to wear a lower denture. Mrs M says that, at about the time she lost her teeth, she was going through the menopause and both sons got married and left home, with the favourite son emigrating. Relations with her husband, never very satisfactory, ceased. The dental incident provided a hook on which she seems to have hung most of the pain of her life's losses – broken glass indeed!

The importance of sexuality

Many elderly people, particularly those who have been long in residential care or who are treated unkindly by their relatives, have a tenuous hold on self-respect. In particular, they may feel they have lost their attractiveness as a man or a woman. It is important to have this recognised and appreciated by some genuinely complimentary remark from the dentist. It can make an enormous difference to an individual's self-esteem to know that his or her appearance and personality can give pleasure.

Slowing down

Advancing age is usually accompanied by physical and mental slowing down. Comprehension may appear to be sluggish and there is an inability to grasp the choices of treatment, but much of this failure of comprehension may be due to hearing or sight loss. Some of us hate wearing spectacles or a hearing aid and will accept the risk of not understanding as long as we do not have to display the outward badges of decay.

If a patient is hard of hearing, there is no point in shouting. The dentist should speak slowly, articulate clearly and let the patient see his mouth. If all else fails, writing it down and, in the case of postoperative instructions, informing the accompanying person, may be necessary.

Increased fragility when submitted to surgical or pharmacological assault

The ability of some older people to withstand any kind of stress is greatly reduced; operative work and lengthy appointments, which would have been quite normal in their younger days, are not well-tolerated. In addition, a longer recovery time should be allowed. Standard adult drug doses may tip a normal elderly person into irrationality, especially if the patient is underweight.

If a patient arrives in a confused state when formerly he had appeared to be quite sensible, his drug history should be carefully checked.

> Mr G, whom the dentist had known and treated for many years, was brought to his surgery because of dental pain. He was quite disorientated and uncooperative. His accompanying daughter said that he had had acute bronchitis and, whilst in hospital, heavy

sedation had been used to control his efforts to get out of bed at night. He had only just returned home. The dentist made an appointment for a week later when the patient had been off all drugs for seven days. He was then rational, sensible and coopera-tive, and treatment was carried out.

'Don't push me about'

An elderly patient has often waited many anxious days or weeks for the visit, thinking and worrying about little else. What is to happen at this encounter will have been mentally rehearsed many times, and the occasion will be extremely important afterwards. To the dentist, however, it will be a brief interview in a busy day. The temptation to deal with the elderly person at the same rate as younger patients must be resisted.

Older patients have an increasing dislike of being hurried or rushed in any way. All procedures should be done slowly and with adequate explanation. To sit an old person in a chair and drop it back to a horizontal position without full explanation can be not only very frightening, but extremely uncomfortable without full neck support.

Many unpleasant things are done to us – either in hospital or in the dental surgery – without time being taken to give a full explanation and achieve understanding, and therefore without our full consent. The need for economy in time often means that dental procedures are carried out on patients who do not completely understand what is being done. A full and proper explanation and informed consent should be given for every procedure, and this is especially important with older and more nervous patients. For example, in the supine position during prolonged dental treatment, some patients are terrified that objects felt in their mouth could go straight down into their lungs. The dentist may not think of explaining that a rubber dam is being used.

Enhanced need for comfort in eating

Elderly people living alone tend to have a restricted diet and, if they have any discomfort in chewing, the diet becomes even more restricted until they become substantially undernourished. The enjoyment of food may be one of the last major sources of pleasure and contentment in old age. In order to enjoy variety in food, comfortable and reasonably efficient teeth are necessary.

A woman went to visit her elderly mother who was usually happy and companionable, but she found her to be extremely fractious and critical, complaining that her teeth were uncomfortable. She found that her mother had been eating nothing but bread soaked in hot water and that all those nourishing single portions of food she had so carefully prepared for her mother's freezer had been left untouched. Her denture problem was happily sorted out, with a marked improvement in her eating, general health and attitudes.

Vanity does not fade with age

We all like to look pleasant and be acceptable in company, whether talking or eating. Loose and clicking dentures can cause older people to withdraw from social contact and become more and more isolated.

A woman, who had a holiday villa in Spain, said recently that when her mother of 85 came to stay with her there, she kept her confined to her room because she made such unpleasant noises with her teeth when eating and her speech was also affected. She did not like being ashamed of her mother before her house guests and so she took the easiest course. A good dentist might have transformed this poor woman's life.

When older people come for dentures, it is important that their appearance is kept substantially the same, not only for prosthetic considerations, but for social reasons as well. A substantial alteration of facial appearance, occasioned by the fitting of new complete dentures, may change relationships with grandchildren and friends for the worse. (See also p. 199.)

In the young, a new look may be exciting, and for publicity-seekers it may increase earning power, but it seldom does much for the elderly.

A patient of 70, who had had extreme loss of hearing from the age of 30, complained bitterly when her husband's odd-shaped mouth had been straightened by a clever dentist and a new set of dentures. She had to learn afresh to lip-read from him.

A district nurse who deals with many old people said that she had seldom seen an attractive denture in an older person. They all seemed to be flat, regular and characterless. She asked whether it was possible for the arrangement and shape of natural teeth to be copied.

We should regard the appearance of the elderly as of similar value to them as our own good appearance is to us.

'No-one listens to what I say'

Some older people have difficulty in articulating, not only because their minds may be slowing down, but because of bad teeth and ill-fitting dentures. Clarity of speech is very important if we are to remain in a social group, and particularly for those who live in residential homes.

If a patient's speech is slow because of a cerebrovascular accident or as part of the slowing-down of great age, the dentist or others may be tempted to end his sentences for him and often do this incorrectly. It is very frustrating not to be given time to express what we want to say, particularly if it will affect what treatment we will receive. Once again, unhurried time to listen to elderly people is important.

FACE-TO-FACE

Some of the points made under the previous headings are of necessity also concerned with the interactions between the dentist's attitudes and the patient's needs. These issues will be further developed in this section, with particular emphasis on transactions that might take place at the first interview.

Approaching patients as unique individuals

Life is easier if we can create stereotypes, categorise and generalise. We can then produce a knee-jerk response when faced by a teenager with a punk hairstyle, or a coloured immigrant, or an elderly person, or a male ballet dancer or a university professor.

An older person who is retired may feel that he has already lost much of his significance, and he is further diminished by attitudes which condescendingly place him in a neat pigeonhole. To address a patient as 'grandad', 'grannie', 'dearie', 'love' or 'sunshine' does not enhance that person's sense of value as an individual. Such expressions as, 'Be a good boy now and keep still', or 'Naughty girl not using your toothbrush', often heard in nursing homes, are positively insulting to those who have physical disabilities but are still mentally active.

We must be able to see beyond the sum of a patient's disabilities and regard each person as uniquely valuable and worthy of respect, no matter what his cleanliness, manner, appearance, disabilities or wealth might be.

The patient needs to feel warmth and respect. This is not communicated by being late, by preoccupation with writing up the last patient's notes, taking a telephone call or being caught washing your hands with your back to him.

He needs to be looked in the eye, addressed by his proper name, welcomed by an appropriate form of bodily contact, to have his health enquired after and the answer waited for! Other persons in the surgery should be introduced to him. He comes in as an insecure patient: he should leave as a friend of the practice.

Talking to the patient

Unless it is quite obvious that he cannot answer for himself, the patient should be spoken to directly and his responses waited for. 'Does he take sugar?' must be a most diminishing way to put the question.

> A spry, elderly widow with a lump in the floor of her mouth was referred by her dentist to an oral surgeon. Her husband's terminal illness had prevented her seeking earlier advice. A biopsy was carried out and she came for the results. The surgeon looked very grave and asked if someone had accompanied her. Her son, who was waiting outside, was brought in and sat opposite to the oral surgeon while the patient was placed at the side. He then explained to the son the gravity of the disease and the treatment that would be necessary. He did not look once at the patient, who was immensely hurt and felt that she was being treated as less than a human being and excluded from taking part in the most important decision of her life.

Was the oral surgeon afraid of an emotional breakdown in the patient if he addressed her directly? Did he not realise she was intelligent and could hear perfectly well? Was he really saying, 'I am a very busy man, this is an old person, the quickest thing I can do is to speak to the son and get on with the next patient'?

Whatever the reason, the result was to destroy any confidence that might have been generated to help her through the next few months.

Communicating without patronising

The patient must be helped to understand what the dentist considers to be the appropriate treatment to meet his particular need. It must be pitched at a level and a speed which makes it quite clear to the patient but does not insult his intelligence. Careful explanation of what may happen after treatment and how the patient has to deal with it must also be given in the same unambiguous manner.

Mr B was slightly mentally affected by his stroke and wondered why the tablet he was given didn't dissolve in water as he had been told it would. The instructions given to him had not included removal of the foil. His hands were very arthritic so that this would have been difficult for him anyway. A short demonstration on how to cut the foil from the tablet, which would have been appropriate for this patient, would have been irritating to another disabled but more alert person.

The dividing line between patronising over-simplicity and not giving enough information can be a narrow one.

A bishop's wife, a vivacious outgoing woman in her late sixties, went to her dentist, who said she needed her last eight teeth removed and would she bring someone with her to hold her hand? There was no discussion on how it would be done or what it would mean. When she arrived, she was given at least ten intraoral injections, and each successive extraction created a sense of mounting horror. It took her a whole year to get over the experience.

The dentist had obviously assumed that his patient was an intelligent person and ought to know about such things, and her bright extrovert personality had concealed the fact that she was fearful. Much more explanation and involvement of the patient herself in the decision might have been helpful.

Standard English

In certain parts of most English-speaking countries there are marked regional accents, different vocabularies and even dialects. Speaking standard English here is no guarantee of being fully understood. Some overseas doctors and dentists may have an additional problem, being under the impression that their English is faultless. This is a common source of complaint by elderly patients. Their professional adviser is a nice man, but what he means is not always plain and there is doubt whether they themselves are always fully understood.

Listening and history-taking

It is important to establish who made the appointment. Did the patient come of his own volition, or was he persuaded to come by a relative or a health worker, or sent by a husband or wife? If the patient has come feeling under some duress, the relationship with the dentist is likely to be more difficult and less fruitful. Sympathetic and kind handling will be essential if the patient's resentment is to be overcome.

The structure and methods of history-taking that we were all taught are commonly abused. The process is often used as a mechanical tool to extract information leading to a diagnosis and treatment plan. The fact is that if we ask questions, we only get answers and these may have nothing to do with the patient's most pressing problems. It is difficult to sit and listen and allow the patient to 'wander', but it is this listening and not asking a barrage of questions which is a valuable way of learning how we can be of most use to the patient.

A simple example is that of an elderly patient who is having discomfort with his dentures. They are old and do not fit very well. As a result of insensitive history-taking, the patient finds himself hustled into having new dentures with all their attendant troubles. He was not really asking for new dentures, he was not asking for a change of appearance; all he really wanted was the comfort of a reline of his favourite 'old slippers'. (See also Chapter 7.)

Attentive listening without too many questions is essential if the patient's real problems are to be understood. He should feel that the dentist is so interested that he can reveal 'stupid' ideas or fantasies which are really worrying. These ideas will never be revealed as answers to questions, and it is essential to give the patient freedom to talk, although this may take up a whole appointment.

An elderly patient revealed one such fantasy when she told the dentist that a barrier had formed in her mouth and that she there-fore could not open it wide enough for dental treatment. The 'barrier' could have symbolised many different things but in this particular patient it was symbolic of a barrier she had built around herself, fearing that anyone who came too close to her would discover that she was worthless. This feeling of worthlessness was rooted in the fact that she was illegitimate and that her legitimate siblings had always had parental preference over her.

The total listening and understanding of the dentist allowed this fantasy to be revealed, discussed and finally resolved so that dental treatment was eventually facilitated.

Total listening means giving eyes, ears and sensitivity to all the verbal and non-verbal communications from the patient so that nothing is missed. We are often distracted from this degree of concentration by thinking what we are going to say next. There does not need to be any immediate response. Silence in conversation can be delightful, and thinking may well be more important than talking.

Use of emotions generated at interview

No patient makes us feel nothing at all. Happiness, satisfaction, pleasure, anxiety, worry, irritation, or other emotions may be experienced, but never nothing. One may feel helpless and uncomfortable with a patient's expression of sadness and grief, or feel defensive and angry at critical demands. These emotions and others should not interfere with listening; they should be valued as clues to be used.

We can respond initially by restating the patient's feelings and their causes, thus making the patient aware that he is being heard by a person who cares and is willing to share his bad feelings.

Emotional responses that patients arouse in the dentist can be used in a constructive manner. A patient may say, 'My daughter excludes me from social occasions because my dentures click and slide about. You fitted these badly two years ago.' A hostile and angry response in return for criticism would be damaging. A helpful reply could be, 'It seems that you are really sad at being left out and you feel the responsibility is with me for not making you better dentures,' and then to allow the patient to enlarge on this. One should never bristle or get angry in return for criticism, but rather encourage patients to talk about their anger and miseries. The objective should be to help the patient to understand the causes of discomfort or resentment.

An elderly patient while visiting her dentist complained of a terrible irritation round and inside her mouth. Her sleep was being disturbed, no ointment or mouthwash she had tried was of any use, and there were no abnormal physical signs. She went on about this until the dentist, who wanted to get on with his day's work, also got irritated. He then suddenly asked himself the meaning of the irritation the patient was conveying to him. When he asked her what the real irritation in her life was, she complained of the way her daughter treated her, never letting her think for herself, never letting her help in the household, always bossing her around and telling her what to do. When the patient realised that this could be the cause of her irritated mouth and lips, she quietly resolved to do something about it. Six months later, she said the irritation had gone. She had moved into a flat of her own, nearby but out of her daughter's house.

Hostile behaviour often conceals underlying anxiety.

An imperious grandfather came to the dentist and in the course of interview demanded that his grandson who had brought him went to the car for his glasses; then he demanded a handkerchief, and finally sent him to make a telephone call. He started asking the young dentist how he could possibly know what the best treatment was. Had he enough experience to carry out the work properly? As the dentist got more and more angry, he looked over and saw the same frustration in the grandson who was a qualified teacher. He suddenly realised that, instead of just swallowing his anger and being frustrated, he could ask the patient whether he felt no satisfactory relationship could be made without one person bossing another. This opened the way for the patient to say how vulnerable he felt as an old man and that if he didn't keep getting on top of everyone, he would lose his grip and sink into anonymity. They then had a conversation about accepting the difficulties of the retired status and the sadness of growing old and losing one's former vigour. By the next visit the patient had settled down, stopped dominating his grandson and the dentist, and the treatment proceeded successfully. The old man felt he had been understood and cared for.

Conversely, pleasant behaviour may conceal a problem.

One old lady smiled very nicely at the dentist and overtly tried to please him, asking after his health although she had never met him before. At the end of treatment she was so grateful to the dentist that he felt rather pleased with himself at doing a good job. The next time she returned it was obvious that what he had done for her had not relieved her symptoms at all but again she was very polite and extremely grateful. He then asked himself, 'Why has this patient got to try to make me feel good when obviously I have not done much for her?' He asked her why she felt it necessary always to keep people happy. She rather sadly told him about the residential home where she lived. Any sign of discontent in the old people meant ostracism by the staff and the deprivation of privileges and so, to survive, she had to put on this face of gratefulness and effort to please. At the next visit the dentist was able to get down to what the patient needed and a much more truthful encounter between them enabled him to plan realistic treatment.

Unconscious communications

An elderly patient who appears in a dirty, untidy condition and with a neglected mouth, who formerly always appeared tidy and clean, is perhaps declaring that life is hardly worth living. Before dental needs are understood and treatment planned, it may be necessary for the dentist to give the patient an opportunity to tell him why life has become so tiresome. To criticise, tolerate or ignore such a communication would be a positive disservice to the patient, and incidentally guarantee the failure of dental treatment.

The patient who approaches the dental chair much more slowly than her arthritis warrants and looks anxious does not need verbal reassurance, but needs to be asked what particularly frightens or upsets her. When the fears have been aired, she is more likely to settle comfortably to treatment.

The bright old person who tells you that he has never been afraid of dentists in his life, and sits in the chair grasping the arms with the whites of his knuckles showing, unconsciously tells another story. If this is not gently commented upon or discussed, he may be even more difficult to treat than the person who admits to fear.

Patients who persistently will not open their mouths fully can be very tiresome, but discussion with such a patient may reveal invasion of other body cavities such as occurs with suppository treatment, catheterisation, or even the use of a colostomy bag. The dental invasion may be just one further insult to the patient's body and a nasty reminder of his failing powers and loss of autonomy and independence. Acknowledgement of his other discomforts may enable him to relax and accept the dental examination and treatment.

Common difficulties sometimes have unique and uncommon origins.

One elderly woman pulled the dentist's hand away when he was

about to give her a local anaesthetic injection. She had been perfectly cooperative up to that moment. She apologised profusely,
lay back, and the dentist began again – and again she pulled his
hand away. This happened several times, thus telling him unconsciously that she had previously suffered some painful intrusion. In
fact, many years earlier she had been assaulted and raped whilst
babysitting and the dentist had unwittingly aroused hidden unconscious fears.

The practice of dentistry involves such a physical closeness
that changes in the level of fear and anxiety are all too easily
picked up. Bland reassurance is often not appropriate, and the
opportunity must be given for the patient to express the cause of
his fears and receive an obvious understanding by the dentist.

The patient who receives the information about treatment
needed with 'I suppose it's my money you're after,' may be
telling you that he has always found it difficult to make trusting
relationships. An accepting, caring attitude is essential here, with
the dentist being able to see the sad person behind the offensive
nature of this communication.

The man who slumps in the chair and says, 'You decide what's
best for me – you're the expert,' may be telling you that he is tired
and is giving up all responsibility for his oral health and reverting
to dependency. If so, such a patient needs gentle encouragement
and regular visits.

Wants and needs

The dentist's view of what is required in treatment may be
entirely at variance with what the patient wants or expects and,
unless there is any urgent, overriding reason in terms of health,
the patient must be left to make an informed choice if he is at all
capable of doing so. To insist that the dentist's particular preference is best further diminishes the patient's area of choice and
responsibility. Many elderly patients want comfort and the least
possible change. They may well, for instance, on losing their few
remaining teeth, refuse to be fitted with dentures.

Mrs D, on the other hand, was incensed when the dentist
proposed removing one of her teeth rather than restoring it, suggesting to her that it would be a lengthy and costly procedure and
she would really be better off at her age to have it removed. As she
still had most of her natural teeth and was careful of her general
health and of her mouth and her appearance, the dentist's dismis-
sive suggestion based on her age quite appalled her.

The management of malignant neoplasms of the jaws in very old people may present great difficulties in knowing what to do for the best. A careful explanation of the various courses of action should be given, and the patient's wishes entirely respected, whether he decides to go forward for treatment or to be left in peace.

Continuing treatment

At the end of the appointment, careful explanation of what has been done should be given, and what is to be expected during the postoperative period. If bruising, swelling or postoperative pain are at all likely, a proper warning and suggestions for management will reduce anxiety and increase confidence. Written postoperative instructions may be even more helpful to the elderly.

Many older patients tend not to want to bother their professional advisers with what might be dismissed as a trivial postoperative symptom. The dentist should make his availability and willingness to see the patient abundantly clear if there is any concern in the postoperative period.

The relationship between patient and dentist is one of intimacy and trust. None of us likes to be handed on to the partner or the assistant, and this feeling is likely to be even stronger in older people. New relationships usually become more and more difficult as age advances. Feelings of disappointment and hostility may be aroused, and much good work done in previous appointments will be undone if the patient is passed to another dentist without the greatest care and for the best of reasons.

POSTSCRIPT

Having insisted that generalisations about older people may be misleading follies, is it now possible to make any worthwhile general points in trying to summarise the messages of this chapter?

Older patients have by definition had a long experience of life and its lessons, and are worthy of great respect. The complexity of this experience has increased rather than diminished their individuality, and a much greater sensitivity is required from professional attendants, together with the devotion of unhurried time.

Insight is essential in all successful human relationships, but this is particularly so with the elderly, where loss and change in many areas are requiring painful adjustment, and where dental treatment may be just one more menace to physical integrity.

In trying to answer the questions, 'What does my patient want, and what does he need?' quiet observation and total listening for all the signals must be achieved.

In recognising and giving thought to the emotions aroused in the dentist by this approach, his understanding of the patient's unarticulated difficulties will become clearer, as will also the recognition of his own emotional and intellectual limitations. Total listening will also accept and consider irrational fantasies about the oral cavity and awaken the realisation that these are often displacements from less acceptable and less easily faced problems.

People are different, elderly people even more so. We owe them our respect, our whole attention, considerable thought, clear communication, and then our best technical skills.

Chapter 2

Ageing in Teeth and Associated Tissues
B. COHEN

AGE CHANGES IN TEETH

The fact that teeth are often the last persisting remains of the human body and that much of our knowledge of prehistoric man is derived from fossil remains of teeth in particular, confers an erroneous impression of their immutability. Curiously, teeth are conspicuously impregnable only after death; during life they are vulnerable to a series of assaults from the days of early development, throughout childhood and into old age. Two major damaging influences are particularly associated with ageing; one is progressive loss of soft-tissue attachments leading to exposure of the root and loosening of teeth within their bony sockets; the second is increasing brittleness that predisposes to cracks, fractures and shearing of tooth substance.

Teeth differ from most other parts of the body in that the regenerative capacity of their constituent tissues is extremely limited. So far as enamel is concerned, passive repair of minor damage by remineralisation has been postulated, but true regeneration is possible only in those teeth of persistent growth seen in certain animal species. Dentine and cementum, unlike enamel, retain a capacity for repair but the formation of reparative dentine inevitably encroaches upon the pulp chamber thus reducing blood supply and drainage, so that, by the time middle age is reached, the vitality of most human teeth is already threatened; three score years and ten is probably a generous estimate for the vitality of the average human tooth pulp.

With regard to the attachment apparatus, each of the constituent tissues is capable of true regeneration but in order for loss of periodontal attachment to be made good integrated repair of epithelium, fibres and cementum would be necessary and such synchrony is not easily contrived (see Fig. 2.4). Moreover, the regenerative capacity of the soft-tissue components is by no means as brisk in old age as in youth. There is evidence from tissue culture experiments to show that cells taken from embryos possess a greater proliferative capacity than those grown from adult tissues and it is a well-known complaint of the elderly (and even of athletes in their thirties!) that injuries take longer to heal than previously.

Various theories have been advanced in attempts to understand the deterioration of structure and function associated with ageing but so far as the teeth are concerned, and certainly in respect of enamel, there is little need to look further than the simple process of wear and tear. So mechanistic an attitude is justifiable only in respect of tissues whose reparative capacity is limited. Even then, regard has to be paid to age changes in associated tissues that can aggravate the degree of wear and tear; for example, diminished secretion from salivary glands, by reducing the beneficial effects of lubrication on masticatory surfaces, could increase the wear sustained by tooth enamel. Incidental though this effect may be, it points to the necessity for considering teeth in relation to their surrounding tissues and to the body as a whole, rather than regarding them in isolation.

Enamel

Attrition, abrasion and erosion are the terms applied to three processes responsible for destroying such enamel as has survived until old age despite the ravages of caries and various other assaults in youth. Loss arising from erosion is not necessarily age-related.

Attrition

This is that form of frictional wear induced during masticatory movements by repeated contact with opposing teeth (occlusal attrition) and adjacent teeth (approximal attrition). Attrition can undoubtedly arise from teeth wearing one another, as is seen in bruxism, but is greatly influenced by the consistency of the diet. Modern foodstuffs are largely free of gritty constituents so that attrition is not now a major cause of tooth loss as it appears to have been in past centuries (Fig. 2.1) and still is in the few remaining primitive societies. An example of the latter is shown in Fig. 2.2; the degree of wear in aborigines is usually attributed to the tough meat and roots they chew but the manner in which they roast their meat probably contributes the abrasive effect of sand and ash to the wear of tooth upon tooth. Marked attrition is seen in Eskimos, who use their teeth not only for the comminution of food but also in the preparation of animal hides; the

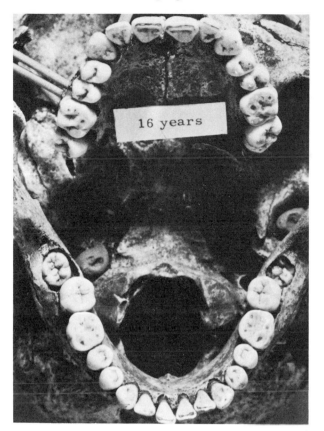

Fig 2.1   *The skull of an Anglo-Saxon who lived about 600 AD. Note that, although the third molars have yet to erupt, marked wear is already evident on the occlusal surfaces of the functional teeth.*

reintroduction of fibre into modern diets could conceivably produce some effect. Patterns of wear should be heeded by clinicians treating other teeth or temporomandibular joint symptoms. To a certain extent it is arguable that attrition is a normal consequence of mastication, but its appearance is also an important indicator of parafunctional activities such as bruxism or pipe-smoking, which take toll of tooth enamel in their different ways. In planning restorative procedures both normal function and idiosyncratic habits have to be allowed for and patterns of attrition often delineate them more accurately than a history elicited from a patient.

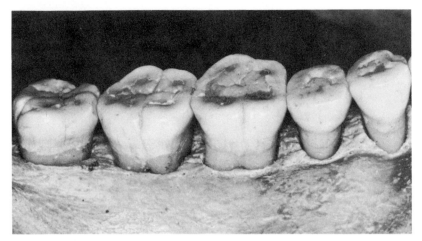

Fig 2.2   *The mandible of an Australian aboriginal. Note the flat occlusal surfaces. The embrasures are broad and the interdental septum of bone appears to be robust.*

Abrasion

This describes the condition in which tooth substance is lost by frictional effects other than those associated with mastication. Damage caused by toothbrushing falls into this category and shows up as transverse scoring of the tooth surface, particularly of canines and premolars, and is usually most marked in the cervical region of crowns on buccal and labial surfaces; it tends to be asymmetrical in its severity, depending upon whether the victim is right- or left-handed. Where gingival recession has occurred, as is usually the case in elderly patients, abrasion of cementum and dentine may be even more marked than that of enamel. At its most severe the degree of abrasion may be such that little force is required to detach the crown from the body of the tooth. Such destruction at the neck of the tooth may be a combined effect of abrasion and erosion.

Erosion

This term designates loss of enamel by the action of ingested or, occasionally, regurgitated acids. Ingested acid excludes that formed on the tooth surface by bacterial fermentation of dietary carbohydrates such as occurs in dental caries. The main source of ingested acid is from citrus fruit; minor sources include vinegar and medication. Normally the consumption of fruit is accompanied by the secretion of saliva, the buffering capacity of which exerts a protective effect. However, the commercial preparation of fruit juices and their consumption in large quantities creates a concentration of acid in the mouth so rapidly that salivary protection, without the adjunct of masticatory cleansing, will inevitably be overcome. Pure lemon juice, the acidity of which (pH 2.2 to 2.4) is little different from that of citric acid, has sometimes been advertised as a slimming aid; whether it confers any benefit in this respect or not is immaterial, because the disastrous effects upon the dentition justify nothing less than a Health Warning on the label of such preparations. According to Weast and Astle (1979) the pH of lime juice (1.8 to 2.0) is even lower than that of lemons; by comparison orange juice (3.0 to 3.4) may appear to be relatively innocuous but it is still far below the pH at which demineralisation of tooth enamel begins – generally agreed to be 5.5. This paper is cited from a comprehensive review of citrus juices and their effects on the teeth by Touyz and Glassman (1981). These authors warned against the increasing consumption of citrus juices – no doubt enhanced by increasingly efficient processing and packaging – and stress that the marketing of these products depends heavily on advertisements extolling the health-promoting properties of vitamin C. Unless the public is made aware of the damaging action on teeth the toll of tooth-loss caused by erosion will become progressively more formidable.

Unlike lesions caused by abrasion, which are characteristically narrow in relation to their depth, areas of erosion are usually saucer-shaped. Moreover, although most commonly seen on the labial surfaces of upper anterior teeth, they are occasionally seen on the lingual aspect of these teeth as well as on occlusal surfaces; in the latter situation concavities may be extensive and this loss is aggravated by chipping away of undermined enamel bordering the eroded concavity as well as by exaggerated wear of exposed dentine.

A distinguishing feature of lesions caused by erosion is that they are more frequently painful than are those resulting from abrasion or attrition. Teeth affected by erosion often become exquisitely sensitive to touch but the exposed dentine can readily be desensitised without recourse to surgical measures.

The management of all these forms of tooth-loss is dealt with in Chapter 6.

The Acquisition of Resistance to Caries. It has long been recognised that coronal dental caries is a disease predominantly of childhood and adolescence. Whether or not the lessening of susceptibility is attributable only to intrinsic change in the composition and structure of tooth enamel is open to question. Certainly there are detectable chemical and physical changes associated with the maturation of enamel. Absorption of fluoride and other ions by surface enamel is a demonstrable phenomenon and passive remineralisation of minor blemishes has already been referred to; many different minerals accumulate in the outer layers of the enamel.

Nevertheless there are several local factors that have been held to account for the diminishing incidence of caries in the elderly. Most obvious is that sites of caries in earlier years have been obliterated, either by tooth-loss or by replacement of lost tooth substance with filling materials. According to this theory the reduced incidence merely reflects a reduction in susceptible sites. Similarly it has been suggested that over the years susceptible sites, especially on occlusal surfaces, come to be greatly reduced by attrition.

A further possible explanation, much less widely espoused than the conventional wisdom mentioned above, is that immunity is acquired to the microorganisms responsible for caries. Proof of this possibility is not easily adduced. Unlike damage arising from most other infections, caries is relatively slow to develop and the presence of cavities in teeth (and certainly of fillings) is not necessarily indicative of current infection but could equally reflect bacterial activity long previously. For this reason the correlation of antibody levels in serum or (less easily) in saliva with caries indices based on the number of decayed, missing and filled teeth, is not one that commands acceptance without reservations. Moreover, even under carefully controlled experimental situations, the precise relationship between antibody levels and caries activity has yet to be established. For all that, it should not be overlooked that, although a diminished number of susceptible sites may contribute to reduced caries in the elderly, the decline in susceptibility after early adult life is consistent with the slow acquisition of immunity to an organism of low immunogenicity.

Dentine

Age changes in dentine are in many ways diametrically different from those seen in enamel. Whereas enamel is incapable of regeneration, new dentine can be laid down for as long as the tooth pulp remains vital although, paradoxically, it infringes upon the pulp chamber and leads, ultimately, towards obliteration of the pulp. The primary dentine laid down in the course of tooth development has a characteristically regular arrangement of dentinal tubules and at the time of tooth eruption it is separated from the pulp by a broad layer of predentine. In the secondary dentine deposited thenceforth the pattern of tubules is much less orderly and, with age, the width of predentine is notably diminished.

Apart from the deposition of secondary dentine two other striking changes occur, namely, the development of dead tracts and of translucent zones. The fact that each of these alterations is so frequently seen to be associated with an overlying carious lesion points to their being protective reactions. The deposition of secondary dentine will clearly serve to protect the delicate pulpal tissue. Translucent zones are presumed to be a similarly protective manifestation. They owe their translucency to the fact that the dentinal tubules of the affected area become occluded by the deposition of mineral salts, the refractive index thus becoming more uniform than that of tubular dentine. These translucent zones, first described by John Tomes more than one hundred years ago, were shown by Fish (1948) to constitute a barrier to the passage of dyes; from this he reasoned that they serve as an impermeable barrier to protect the pulp from toxic substances.

It is relevant to mention that translucent zones commonly occur within the root dentine of the elderly. They are, in fact, so regularly seen that they provide a useful indicator when age has to be assessed for forensic purposes. Miles (1976) provides details of this and many other age changes in teeth.

When translucent zones develop beneath carious lesions they are usually associated with the type of lesion that progresses only slowly. Where destruction occurs more rapidly the dentinal response is usually in the form of what Fish (1948) described as a dead tract. Here the dentine is more than normally opaque and, as in translucent zones, the odontoblast and its process have been lost but, contrary to what occurs in translucent zones, the tubules remain empty and it is this that confers their relative opacity when transilluminated. Although dead tracts and translucent zones appear in most instances to have been a response to noxious external stimuli (such as caries or attrition) both are sometimes found in teeth that have remained unerupted; this suggests that to some extent the sealing of dentinal tubules is also a change associated with the ageing process.

Pulp

The principal age change in the tooth pulp is that the chamber and canals it occupies become progressively reduced in size by the deposition of secondary dentine. Other forms of calcification are also common but the causes underlying the formation of dysplastic mineralised tissue, often in concentrically laminated masses known as pulp stones, are undefined.

With age the pulp becomes less cellular, less vascular and more fibrous. Recent work (Fried and Erdelyi 1984) has shown that major changes can be seen in teased pulpal nerve fibres in cats. Both the length and the diameter of fibres are substantially reduced with age and qualitative changes, including evidence of demyelination, are commonly observed. In the light of these findings it is not surprising that the sensitivity of dentine decreases in the elderly. As mentioned above, the width of predentine is gradually reduced and the odontoblasts that line its pulpal aspects are not only less numerous but are also shrunken in appearance. Following a successful partial pulpectomy a bridge of dentine comes to cover the exposed pulp, so that regeneration of the odontoblast layer, possibly from a reserve of undifferentiated pulp cells, is a demonstrable phenomenon. For a detailed description of the pulp-dentine complex the reader is referred to Miles (1976) and to Symons (1976).

Apart from the diminution in size of the pulp chamber and canals, ageing is also associated with a gradual diminution in the diameter of the apical foramen. It is this that may well account for the progressive loss of vascularity, a change that could conceivably explain most of the degenerative changes seen in elderly pulps.

Cementum

Like dentine, cementum is gradually deposited throughout life and this is the principal cause of narrowing of the apical foramen.

There is clear evidence to suggest that the deposition of cementum can be provoked by external stimuli and it is presumably a succession of low-grade insults over many years that accounts for the relative frequency of hypercementosis in elderly teeth. When this is particularly prominent at the root apex a ball and socket arrangement results, and this leads to difficulty in extracting teeth without fracturing their roots.

Root caries

Cavitation on the root surface differs in many respects from dental caries that starts in enamel. It is seen predominantly in the elderly because extensive areas of the tooth root are rarely exposed in earlier years. Whereas in coronal caries vertical penetration characteristically precedes lateral extension, the lesion in root caries is usually broad and shallow. It is not surprising that the pattern of decay in cementum should differ from that occurring in the much more highly mineralised enamel and, although the pathogenesis of root caries is not precisely understood, there is evidence that actinomycetes rather than streptococci are likely to be the principal causative organisms. The shape of the root, the site of the lesion and the structure of cementum are all so different from the features prevailing in enamel caries that the restorative dentist is confronted by an entirely different set of problems in the treatment of root caries (see Chapter 6), and prevention of these lesions commands high priority in treatment planning for elderly patients.

Once cementum has become exposed to contamination by food and mouth bacteria it is particularly important that time and care should be devoted to scrupulous maintenance of oral hygiene. It has to be borne in mind, however, that cementum is far less resistant to mechanical injury than is enamel, and vigorous brushing or the use of firm toothbrushes can be expected to result in damage no less undesirable than root caries. It has to be remembered, too, that once cementum becomes exposed the best that can be hoped for is to arrest the process of recession; hence the initiation of procedures to protect the cementum calls for patience on the part of the dentist and perseverance on the part of the patient. A regime of home care has to be devised to enable the patient to reach and to clean areas that, without instruction and practice, would seem to be inaccessible; apart from providing instruction and encouragement the dentist can assist by the application of agents designed to harden or otherwise strengthen the exposed cementum. Various fluoride preparations, excluding acidified gels, are likely to be useful for this purpose.

AGE CHANGES IN THE PERIODONTIUM

Bone

In the developmental years, bone is a conspicuously labile tissue. Resorption and deposition occur synchronously in the process of growth and remodelling. This phenomenon is essential for achieving a balance between structure and function for it is the latter that influences the fine detail of bone development within the broad limits set by genetic influence and metabolic considerations.

With maturity, and once growth is complete, bone is notably less labile although homeostatic regulation necessitates some degree of continuing resorption and deposition. As physical activity diminishes, so too does the demand for new bone formation and, by the time old age is reached, atrophy has resulted

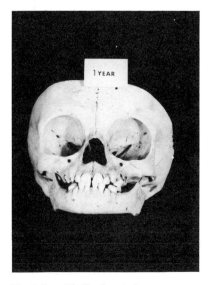

Fig 2.3a   *Skull of an infant.*

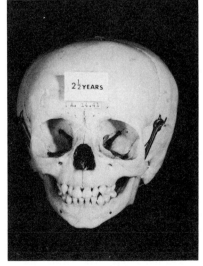

Fig 2.3b   *Skull of a child.*

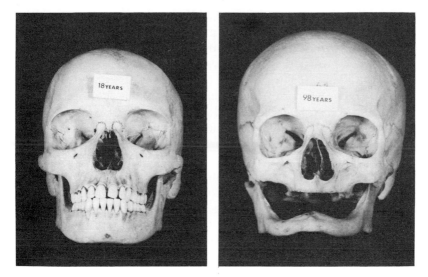

Fig 2.3c   *Skull of an adult.*   Fig 2.3d   *Skull of a geriatric adult.*

from slow resorption that has not been compensated for. The skulls of an infant, a child, an adult and an old man (Figs 2.3a–d) exemplify the changing flux in bone formation; their appearance also provides a reminder of the dangers inherent in extracting teeth or buried root fragments in elderly patients and emphasises the difficulties confronting the prosthodontist.

Increasing fragility is not merely a consequence of atrophy. In addition, the composition of bone gradually alters, resulting in reduced resilience and increased brittleness. It has been estimated that the mineral content of vertebral bone has been reduced by 50% in normal women by the age of 75 years; the comparable figure for men is a 40% decrease (Genant et al., 1983). At a microscopic level it is noteworthy that the cellular component diminishes progressively as age advances, so that the bone appears to be sclerotic and the surviving osteocytes shrunken. Above all, however, the quantity of mineralised tissue is conspicuously reduced, with both cortical and trabecular bone affected.

Periodontal attachment

Loss of the alveolar bone that normally surrounds tooth roots and affords anchorage for the fibres of the periodontal ligament is hastened by the extraction of teeth. Before then this bone resorbs slowly (while the level of the gingiva also recedes) but more rapidly, and irregularly, in the presence of periodontal disease. Just where to draw the line between physiological recession and periodontal disease is a problem that confounds epidemiologists and has given rise to a variety of ingenious but as yet not infallible scoring systems. There is little doubt that figures suggesting the universal prevalence of periodontal disease are inflated by the inclusion of data reflecting changes in the periodontal tissues inseparable from the process of getting older. Analogously, it could certainly be said that alopecia of varying forms is a pathological condition, but records of its incidence would be seriously distorted by including all cases of baldness.

No dentist can enjoy an understanding of periodontal health or disease without a full appreciation of the events underlying gingival recession. This alone justifies reiterating an oft-told series of events. Before a tooth erupts into the mouth it is cocooned in an envelope of odontogenic epithelium. The first cusp to peep through the oral mucosa has breached both the odontogenic epithelium and the epithelial surface of the oral mucosa. The two epithelia merge as they retract and so come to encircle the tooth in a tight cuff – just as a surgical glove would if penetrated by a finger tip. As more and more of the tooth emerges so does the junctional epithelium recede towards the cement–enamel boundary. By virtue of its unique ability to attach at both the connective tissue and tooth interfaces, junctional epithelium is able to constitute a seal that protects the connective tissue of the periodontium from the oral environment. In perfect periodontal health the apical extremity of this seal would be located at the cement–enamel junction when eruption is complete.

Inevitably the seal will be breached, either in the course of mastication by the shearing effect of even minor movement of teeth or as a consequence of mechanical injury such as might be caused by sharp particles of food. As soon as the most coronal attachment of fibre to cementum is disrupted, repair can be effected by renewal of the seal at a level slightly apical to the cement–enamel boundary. The junctional epithelium, which seals the crevice by its adhesion to the root surface, does possess the capacity to regenerate and, with repeated wear and tear, it assumes a progressively more apical attachment. This is illustrated in Fig. 2.4. It is noteworthy that the slender strands of epithelial cells that encircle the tooth, known as the debris of

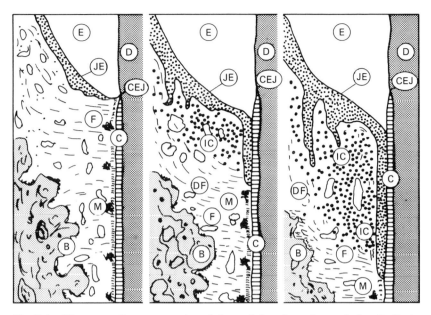

Fig 2.1   *Diagrammatic representation of the periodontal attachment in longitudinal section.*

Left
In perfect health the apical extremity of the junctional epithelium is located at the cement–enamel junction.

Centre
After the loss of the superficial part of the periodontal attachment, the denuded area is repaired by a downgrowth of junctional epithelium; the crest of the alveolar bone is reduced and more of the tooth is exposed.

Right
This depicts the appearance in advanced periodontal disease. Bone has receded, much of the periodontal attachment has been destroyed, progressively more of the cementum is exposed and junctional epithelium extends along the root surface unless interrupted by the inflammatory infiltration.

E = Enamel; D = Dentine; JE = Junctional epithelium; F = Fibres; CEJ = Cement–enamel junction; C = Cementum; IC = Inflammatory cells; DF = Disintegrating fibres; M = Rests of Malassez; B = Bone

Malassez, have been observed to undergo proliferation in response to injury; clearly they are not mere odontogenic flotsam as they were once thought to be and could constitute a reserve of epithelial cells available for providing a new seal as the gingivae recede. In section, the strands appear as small islands of epithelium and Reeve (1960) observed that they decrease in number with age.

The further the gingival margin recedes, the more the tooth root becomes exposed and the more the attachment apparatus is weakened. How is the clinician to determine whether this is a truly pathological change or whether it is merely indicative of natural wear and tear? In elderly patients the distinction is not always obvious. As a general rule, however, wear and tear produces uniform and symmetrical rather than irregular recession and, because this type of recession is relatively slow, loss of periodontal attachment is compensated for by additional deposition of cementum and increased content of collagen in the ligament. For these reasons, well-worn teeth with advanced recession are often surprisingly firm – as the inexperienced exodontist may learn to his cost. Mobility and gingival bleeding are seen only when periodontal disease proper has become established.

Whether the loss of attachment is a result of physiological recession or a pathological process, impaired oral hygiene is a consequence to be avoided. In its early stages recession may in fact facilitate the cleansing of approximal tissues but patients should receive careful instruction on the damage that can be done by misguided toothbrushing; the 'towelling method' described in Chapter 7 is recommended as a safe and efficacious alternative.

CHANGES IN THE ORAL MUCOSA

The oral mucosa possesses no singular feature to make it any more or any less susceptible to the effects of ageing. Much of what is seen as a gradual deterioration in bodily efficiency has a central origin – for example, increasing cardiac insufficiency inevitably affects the vascularity of all tissues, or the gradual involution of ductless glands is accompanied by diminished hormonal stimuli.

The wrinkling of facial skin is matched by a less obvious slow atrophy and loss of the oral mucosa. Comparison with an ageing apple is apposite: the shrivelling of skin and shrinkage of the inner substance reflect the drying out of the juice within. Elderly patients suffer a loss of tissue fluid associated with reduced vascularity, but dryness of the surface also results from reduced secretion of saliva. This depletion is attributable to an age-related decrease in acinar tissue as compared with ductal and connective tissue. These and other features were reported by Waterhouse et al., (1973) and Scott (1977) from examination of major salivary glands, and latterly by Drummond and Chisholm (1984) from a study of ageing effects in labial minor glands. These findings are compatible with the degenerative changes seen in experiments where the duct of a major gland is ligated.

Dryness of the mouth and shrinkage of the soft tissues have far-reaching implications for the clinician treating the elderly. These patients are deprived of the protection afforded by salivary secretions so that their tissues become increasingly vulnerable to minor injury. Reference is made to some of the consequences and to their alleviation in Chapter 3.

Wound healing, a conspicuously successful process in the oral mucosa, becomes progressively less rapid with advancing age. Several different factors contribute to this state of affairs. Vascularity, as already mentioned, diminishes with diminished cardiac output but also as a consequence of impaired haemodynamics locally, arising from damage to and thickening of vessel walls; depletion of the immune response adds to the problems of superimposed infection; and, by no means least, the capacity of cells to undergo division declines to the point where the proliferative response essential to repair is deficient.

MUSCLES AND THE TEMPOROMANDIBULAR JOINT

In common with other soft tissues already discussed, muscles waste as old age approaches. The fibres decrease in size as well as in number, being replaced by fat and fibrous connective tissue. So far as the muscles of mastication are concerned, wastage is no doubt due in part to disuse; less and less muscular effort is required, either because of a failing dentition or a progressively softer diet or, as is often the case, both. (Lewis Carroll invoked poetic licence when he said that the old man who devoured a goose had developed lifelong masticatory power by arguing with his wife.)

The dwindling power of the muscles of mastication is much less likely to cause problems than is degenerative change in the temporomandibular articulation. Temporomandibular dysfunction is by no means confined to the elderly and the literature is heavily slanted towards its occurrence in young subjects, but evidence of age-related disease in the mandibular joint is sufficient to warrant its consideration when masticatory problems arise in old people. In a review of epidemiological studies Helkimo (1976) found that symptoms of mandibular dysfunction are more frequent in the old than the young. Osterberg and Carlsson (1979) studied 30% of all 70-year-olds in Gothenburg, and 384 subjects were subjected to a comprehensive dental examination with a view to assessing masticatory function. Nearly half suffered severe dysfunction; in more than half the masticatory muscles were tender; and in more than one-third abnormal joint sounds could be elicited. Finally, Toller and Glynn (1976), in a study of 150 cases of degenerative disease of the mandibular joint, found that the mean age of patients with osteoarthrosis involving the upper joint cavity was 62 years.

REFERENCES

Drummond J. R., Chisholm D. M. (1984). A qualitative and quantitative study of the ageing human labial salivary glands. *Arch. Oral. Biol.*; **29**: 151–5.

Fish E. W. (1948). *Surgical Pathology of the Mouth*. London: Pitman and Sons.

Fried K., Erdelyi G. (1984). Changes with age in canine tooth pulp-nerve fibres of the cat. *Arch. Oral. Biol.*; **29**: 581–5.

Genant H. K., Cann C. E., Pozzi-Mucelli R. F., Canter A. S. (1983). Vertebral mineral determination by quantitative computerised tomography. *J. Comp. Ass. Tomography*; **7**: 554.

Helkimo M. (1976). Epidemiological surveys of dysfunction of the masticatory system. *Oral Sciences Reviews*; **7**: 54–66.

Miles A. E. W. (1976). Age changes in dental tissues. In *Scientific Foundations of Dentistry* (Cohen B., Kramer I. R. H., eds.) pp. 435–50. London: William Heinemann Medical Books.

Osterberg T., Carlsson G. E. (1979). Symptoms and signs of mandibular dysfunction in 70-year-old men and women in Gothenburg, Sweden. *Community Dental Oral Epidemiol.*; **7**: 315–21.

Reeve C. M. (1960). Epithelial rests in the periodontal ligament of humans. *J. Dent. Res.*; **39**: 746.

Scott J. (1977). Quantitative age changes in the histological structure of human submandibular salivary glands. *Arch. Oral Biol.*; **22**: 221–7.

Symons N. B. B. (1976). Dentine and pulp. In *Scientific Foundations of Dentistry* (Cohen B., Kramer I. R. H., eds.) pp. 423–33. London: William Heinemann Medical Books.

Toller P. A., Glynn L. E. (1976). Degenerative disease of the mandibular joint. In *Scientific Foundations of Dentistry* (Cohen B., Kramer I. R. H., eds.) pp. 725–34. London: William Heinemann Medical Books.

Touyz L. Z., Glassman R. M. (1981). Citrus, acid and teeth. *J. Dent. Assoc. of South Africa*; **36**: 195–201.

Waterhouse J. P., Chisholm D. M., Winter R. B., Patel M., Yale R. S. (1973). Replacement of functional parenchymal cells by fat and connective tissue in human submandibular salivary glands: an age-related change. *J. Oral Pathol.*; **2**: 16–27.

Weast R. C., Astle M. J. (1979). Approximate pH values. In *Handbook of Chemistry and Physics*, 60th edn. pp. D187. Chemical Rubber Company.

Chapter 3 ———————————————————

Oral Mucosal Disease in the Elderly

W. H. BINNIE and J. M. WRIGHT

Oral mucosal diseases become more prevalent with advancing age due to a variety of factors. These include age changes in the mucosal tissues, reduced salivary flow, reduced immunological competence, increased prevalence of systemic diseases and the increased likelihood of therapeutic drug use.

ORAL CANCER

While it may be unusual to begin a discussion of diseases of the oral mucosa in the elderly with neoplasia, oral cancer is not only the most serious disease encountered but is directly age-related. In order to understand the extent and nature of the problem, it may be helpful to look at some facts and figures.

Malignant neoplasms of the oral tissues are rare in the western world when compared with such sites as lung, stomach, colon, rectum, breast, uterus, and skin. They account for only 2% of all malignant tumours. The vast majority (estimated at 90%) are squamous cell carcinomas, the remainder being predominantly malignant tumours of minor salivary gland tissue and (rarely) lymphomas, sarcomas, and melanomas. In the United Kingdom, for example, approximately 2400 cases are registered each year and the number of deaths annually is half the number of new cases. So, although the incidence is small, it is a highly lethal disease and even curable cases may be severely mutilating.

The lower lip is the most common site for squamous cell carcinoma to develop and this is followed by tongue (lateral and ventral surfaces), floor of mouth, alveolar ridge, and buccal mucosa. The hard palate and upper lip are rarely involved and neoplasms of these sites usually originate from minor mucous glands and not from surface epithelium.

The disease is three times more common in men than in women, a ratio which is not as high as it used to be. There has been a slow but steady decline in incidence in the white male population of the United Kingdom and the United States over the last three or four decades whereas the incidence in women has stayed the same throughout the same period. It is important to keep this in mind when examining aetiological factors.

Oral cancer is very much an age-related disease. Ninety-eight per cent of cases occur in persons over the age of 40. The overall incidence in the population is only one in 20 000 but this changes to one in approximately 1100 of the 75 and over male population. The elderly are, therefore, the population group at risk and it is obviously important that dentists carefully examine the oral mucosa of their elderly patients.

Aetiological factors

Since the early part of this century (Power 1918) there has evolved a traditional list of factors associated with the development of oral cancer. These include tobacco, alcohol, syphilis, dental sepsis, and iron deficiency and – although large numbers of studies have been done that have resulted in volumes of print – the evidence is still equivocal. More recently chronic candidiasis and viral infection have been added to the list of related factors. It is beyond the scope of this chapter to review all the information, and the interested reader is referred to an article by Binnie et al. (1983). An attempt, however, to summarise current thinking will be given here.

There is little disagreement about the causative factors of squamous cell carcinoma of the lower lip. Like cancer of the facial skin there is a direct relationship with exposure to actinic radiation. The disease is uncommon in blacks, it is more common in the white population in high sunlight areas, and the prevalence is higher in those with outdoor occupations. In addition to sunlight, it is generally agreed that pipe smoking is also related (Levin et al. 1950, Wynder et al. 1957).

Unfortunately, intraoral carcinogenesis is not as clear-cut and it is important to look at the aetiological factors both individually and in combination.

Tobacco

Tobacco is basically used in two ways, burned and unburned. There is no question that there is a positive relationship between oral cancer and the use of topical tobacco in the form of snuff or chewing tobacco. Not only is the incidence many times higher in areas such as India and the Southeastern United States where the habit is prevalent, but the cancer which develops is site-related, i.e. the carcinoma develops where the tobacco is habitually held (Mahboubi 1977, Waldron 1970). Recently, in response to the dramatic increase in total production of smokeless tobacco in the United States, Winn et al. (1981) reported a four-fold increase in the risk of oral and pharyngeal cancer and a fifty-fold increase for carcinoma of the gingiva and buccal mucosa in a predominantly female population of long-term users in the United States.

If one looks at smoking in isolation, i.e. disassociating other factors, there is a mild increase in risk of developing intraoral cancer, particularly of the tongue and floor of the mouth (Doll and Hill 1964, Rothman and Keller 1972) but the risk is greater for pipe and cigar smokers than for cigarette smokers (Wynder et al. 1957). Since the disease has been steadily declining in incidence, this parallels the trend in consumption of pipe and cigar tobacco (Fig. 3.1). As can be seen, cigar and pipe tobacco consumption has been decreasing whereas cigarette consumption has been increasing until relatively recently.

Alcohol

The evidence implicating alcohol in the development of oral cancer has been confusing, and one of the most commonly cited reasons for the lack of definitive evidence on the carcinogenic capacity of alcohol is the difficulty of isolating heavy alcohol consumption from smoking. Nevertheless, there are studies which do show a positive relationship when controlled for smoking (Schwartz et al. 1962, Rothman 1978, Mashberg et al. 1981). The question which then arises is whether this is due to direct effects of ethanol or other products of the distillation process. It is interesting to note that Massé (1972) demonstrated that by far the highest incidence of oesophageal cancer (which parallels oral cancer) in France is found in the apple-growing areas of Brittany and Normandy. Not only is this incidence the highest in Europe but it is increasing. Although he considered many possible aetiological agents, the associated factor turned out to be a crude home-distilled 'calvados'. Another study contrasting oral cancer in Puerto Rico with the mainland United States (Fischman and Martinez 1977) suggested that the prevalence of home-processed rum might in part account for the higher incidence reported in Puerto Rico. It should also be noted that a link between a high level of alcohol consumption, liver cirrhosis and oral cancer has

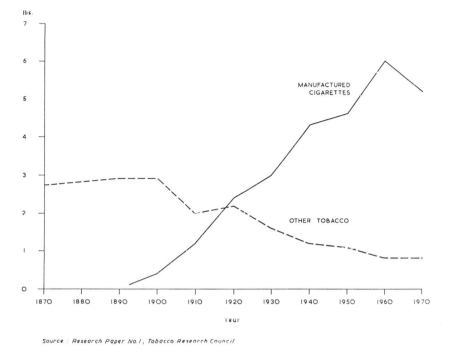

Source : *Research Paper No.1, Tobacco Research Council*

Fig 3.1 *Tobacco consumption in UK (lb per adult).*

been documented by several authors (Trieger et al. 1958, Martinez 1969). It is possible that the liver dysfunction and nutritional deficiency associated with high alcohol consumption may produce predisposition to carcinoma rather than alcohol being a primary carcinogen.

Finally, it must be remembered that the incidence of oral cancer is decreasing, while this is certainly not the case with alcohol consumption in the United Kingdom (Fig. 3.2). It is highly unlikely, therefore, that ethanol produced under government control in the United Kingdom is carcinogenic.

Although the evidence for smoking and alcohol may be conflicting, there is strong evidence to suggest that there is a synergistic effect when both habits occur together. In fact Rothman (1978) has shown that joint exposure results in risk ratios two-and-a-half times that expected if the risk were merely additive. Heavy smokers who are also heavy drinkers have a risk ratio 15 to 20 times higher than nonsmokers and nondrinkers.

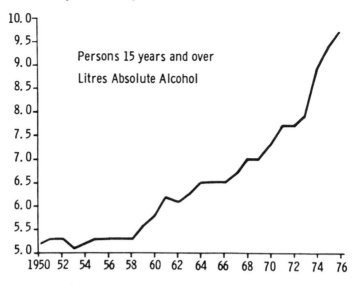

Fig 3.2   *UK annual per capita alcohol consumption.*

Iron deficiency

Iron metabolism is important in maintaining the health of the oral mucosa (Rennie et al. 1984). Many diseased states are associated with iron depletion. Since 1919, when Kelly and Paterson independently described the syndrome that bears their name, it has been known that squamous cell carcinoma of the upper gastrointestinal tract shows a higher incidence in patients who are chronically iron deficient. The mechanisms are not fully understood, and it may well be that iron deficiency is not a primary but a secondary factor in malignant transformation of the oral epithelium. Significant alterations in the immune response occur in iron deficient patients and, as Joynson et al. (1972) have remarked, 'this condition carries important implications with regard to the pathogenesis of malignant disease and chronic infections such as candidiasis.' Iron deficiency is said to be the most common deficiency disease in the world and evaluation (and correction if necessary) of iron status is probably a useful preventive measure in elderly patients. (See p. 104 et seq.)

Syphilis

Infectious agents such as those causing syphilis, chronic candidiasis and herpetic infections have associations with oral cancer. The long-standing strong association between syphilis and tongue cancer is still unclear and likely to remain so. It may well be that substances used in the treatment of syphilis before the use of antibiotics, such as arsenicals and heavy metals, were more influential as carcinogenic agents than the infective organism itself. However, there has been no evidence that the widespread introduction of antibiotic therapy has been accompanied by a sharp decrease in oral cancer.

Candidiasis

Candidal hyphae found in the surface layers of dysplastic oral epithelium have traditionally been assumed to represent a superimposed infection, but this concept has recently been challenged by Cawson and Binnie (1980). In their view there is circumstantial evidence that chronic hyperplastic candidiasis precedes the development of epithelial dysplasia. Further evidence is required before a positive relationship can be established, and other factors such as iron deficiency and immune status must be examined.

Herpes virus

Since 1968, when Rawles et al. reported that women with cervical cancer had high antibody titres to Herpes Simplex Virus type II (HSV-II), many investigators have looked for a similar relationship between HSV-I and oral cancers. So far, there is no evidence of a direct causative relationship, but immunological changes associated with HSV and cancer patients have been reported (Smith et al. 1976). Shillitoe (1982) concluded from his studies that there was a role for HSV-I in the pathogenesis of oral cancer, and suggested that the tumour results from interactions between the virus and tobacco smoke. Currently, speculation has arisen about the possible role of Human Papilloma Virus (HPV) because of the accumulating evidence linking it with cancer of the vagina and uterine cervix.

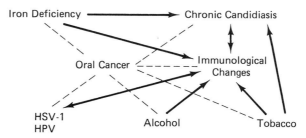

Fig 3.3   *Diagram showing relation of known risk factors for oral cancer (dotted lines) and the effect these factors have on each other (solid lines).*

Dental disease

Chronic neglect of the teeth and periodontal tissues has long been considered an important predisposing or exciting factor in the development of oral cancer. Although studies have shown a high incidence of oral neglect in cancer patients, they do not provide evidence for a cause-and-effect relationship as this would be difficult to estimate retrospectively with any degree of accuracy. However, without definite evidence, there is a commonly held belief among cancer therapists that the decrease in oral cancer incidence is due to improved dental health. This may be true, and certain dental factors may potentiate the development of oral cancer, but at the present time there is little evidence to link the two. On the other hand, it must be stated that neither is there evidence to disprove the association.

Despite all the accumulated data it will be obvious to the reader that there is still no single environmental factor, the removal of which would abolish the disease. The cause of oral cancer is multifactorial and many of the implicated factors are interlinked (see Fig. 3.3). It must be concluded therefore that since we cannot positively reduce the incidence of the disease in our elderly patients, the emphasis must be on reducing mortality, morbidity and mutilation by early diagnosis and institution of appropriate therapy.

Clinical features

Most clinicians are aware of the clinical appearance of an advanced or late-stage squamous cell carcinoma and have little difficulty in establishing the diagnosis. These lesions are either exophytic or invasive and destructive. The exophytic lesion is usually a broad-based, elevated mass with a rough nodular or warty surface. It is indurated at its base and margins and, as the tumour becomes more bulky, necrosis may develop so that the central area becomes ulcerated. The advanced destructive lesion is indurated and shows a classical crater-like defect with raised rolled margins.

It is the early cancer (or precancerous lesion) that is the important one to recognise because it is at this stage that the patient has the greatest chance for cure with minimal morbidity. Unfortunately, the clinical features of early lesions are highly variable, may appear deceptively innocent, and may simulate other oral mucosal conditions. The early lesion may appear as a white patch (leukoplakia) (Fig. 3.4), a velvety red patch (erythroplakia), a small polypoid mass, or a shallow ulcer. The *only* way to determine the nature of these early lesions is by histological investigation, but unfortunately biopsy is often only performed by those clinicians who have a keen understanding of the cancerous process and who maintain a high level of suspicion for mucosal changes. In general, any lesion in the mouth for which a cause cannot be found or which does not resolve within two weeks either spontaneously or after its apparent cause has been

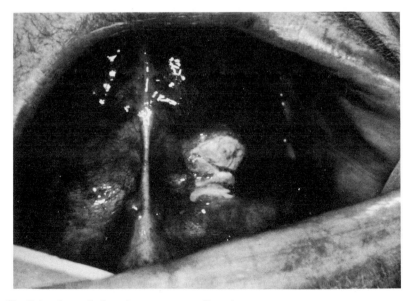

Fig 3.4 *An early invasive squamous cell carcinoma.*

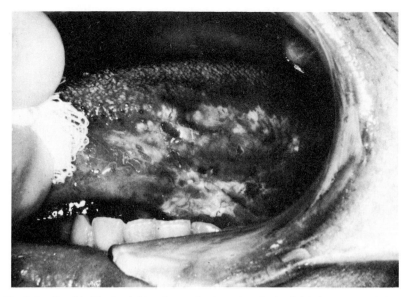

Fig 3.5   *Speckled leukoplakia. Areas of redness in a leukoplakia have more sinister implications. Biopsy showed this to be carcinoma-in-situ.*

removed, should be considered cancerous until biopsy proves otherwise.

Precancerous lesions (dysplastic but not invasive) and early cancerous lesions usually manifest a colour change that can be detected clinically as leukoplakia or erythroplakia. Of all intra-oral leukoplakias from all sites, roughly 20% will prove to be premalignant or malignant when first biopsied (Waldron and Shafer 1975). It is known that certain clinical changes within a leukoplakia reflect a greater likelihood that it is sinister. Those changes include areas of redness (Fig. 3.5), areas of nodularity, or areas with a verrucous surface (Axell et al. 1984). Further-more, leukoplakias in certain intraoral sites carry a higher risk. These include the floor of the mouth, lateral border of the tongue, and lower lip. Erythoplakias are less common than leukoplakias but most will prove to be precancerous or cancer-ous when biopsied. Most early asymptomatic cancers are red rather than white and, in one study, 86% of early oral cancers were predominantly red (Mashberg 1978). Erythroplakias are found most commonly in the floor of the mouth, ventral and lateral borders of the tongue, and soft palate (Mashberg and Meyers 1976).

Carcinoma of the lip

The vast majority of squamous cell carcinomas of the lip involve the lower lip and in fact the few cancers that occur on the upper lip usually originate in minor salivary glands. Lower lip cancers most often develop on the vermilion border approximately half way between the midline and commissure. The early lesion usually appears as a localised thickened area which may have a white or crusted covering and the patient may have thought that this was a cold sore (herpes labialis) which persisted rather than healed. Like skin cancer, lip lesions seldom arise on otherwise healthy-looking tissue. Solar changes such as elastosis, keratosis, irregular pigmentation, telangiectasia and chronic fissures, as well as a lack of clear-cut definition between the vermilion border and skin, are usually features preceding or associated with the development of malignancy.

Although lip cancers are obvious and usually grow slowly they will, if ignored, inevitably develop into a large ulcerating mass with extensive invasion of the musculature of the lip. Metastases, though later to develop and less frequent than from intraoral sites, do occur and then the submental and submandibular lymph nodes are the chief sites of involvement.

Intraoral cancer

Carcinoma of the tongue is less common than that of the lip but it is by far the most common intraoral site. In contrast to lip cancer it is a highly lethal disease and the prognosis for advanced lesions is exceedingly poor. This is a condition in which the dentist may play a critical role in early detection and so provide the only possible hope of cure. In the early stages the lesion is usually asymptomatic and careful examination of the tongue is necessary for detection. The most commonly involved areas are the lateral border near the junction of the anterior and posterior junction and the ventral surface. Primary lesions of the dorsum are exceedingly rare and in the past have been particularly associated with syphilitic glossitis. The initial appearance may be an area of local thickening or roughness, a white patch, or an area of superficial ulceration or erosion. Advanced carcinomas of the tongue tend to be deeply invasive and the whole substance of the tongue musculature may become immobilised, resulting in difficulty with speech, dysphagia and severe pain. Lesions metastasise early to the regional lymph nodes (possibly involving the contralateral side) and the first sign of lingual cancer may be a lump in the neck.

The floor of the mouth is another important primary site for oral cancer, and like the tongue, has a poor prognosis. The advanced lesion may be exophytic or ulcerative but the early lesion may well appear simply as an innocuous-looking red patch (erythroplakia), white patch (leukoplakia) or speckled erythroplakia. It cannot be over-stressed how sinister some of these apparently innocuous lesions may be when found in the floor of the mouth. On biopsy they may turn out to be benign, but in this site the following points are worth remembering. The vast majority of speckled lesions turn out to be carcinoma or severe epithelial dysplasia. Secondly, it is known that a high percentage of the white lesions in this site, termed 'sublingual keratoses' by Kramer et al., (1978), will eventually become malignant. These lesions are bilaterally symmetrical with a well-defined margin, they may well be histologically benign for years, and were thought to be benign developmental naevi (Cooke 1956). There is no doubt, however, that if any change in appearance occurs it has serious implications.

Other intraoral sites are less common but squamous cell carcinoma does develop on the gingival and alveolar mucosa, buccal mucosa and sulcus. It should be remembered, however, that in those regions where the tobacco-chewing habit is common these are much more frequently the sites of squamous cell carcinoma. Gingival lesions tend to be exophytic and may resemble hyperplastic gingivitis, but it has been shown by Panagopoulos (1959) that there is a high incidence of microscopic bone invasion despite negative radiographic findings. These areas of the mouth are the sites of involvement of verrucous carcinoma, which should be thought of as a specific clinicopathological entity. This is a warty, superficially spreading, exceedingly well-differentiated form of squamous cell carcinoma. It has the best prognosis of all oral malignancies in that invasion and metastases rarely develop and, when they do, this occurs at a late stage in the disease. Verrucous carcinoma is most common in areas where there is an associated tobacco-chewing habit but does occur, although rarely, without tobacco use.

Treatment and prognosis

Diagnosis and institution of treatment must occur as early as possible in order to achieve a reasonable chance of cure. Surgical excision, radiotherapy and chemotherapy may be used singly or in combination although chemotherapy on its own would only be used for palliation and not as an attempt at cure. Treatment regimens vary and depend on the site and stage of the disease. If a lesion is small (e.g. less than 2cm), localised and accessible, then surgical excision with clear margins may be sufficient to effect a cure. If the lesion is more extensive and/or local lymph node involvement is suspected, more radical excision with neck dissection would be required, possibly combined with radiotherapy, chemotherapy, or both. Radiotherapy or chemotherapy may be employed before or after surgery. When planning treatment, it is obviously important to consider the age and physical status of the patient in order to determine the degree of possible impairment to quality of life.

If the oral tissues are to be irradiated it is exceedingly important that all dental sepsis be removed, and this may involve full clearance of teeth. Therapeutic radiation by implantation, megavoltage transmission, or radioactive isotopes such as cobalt produces ischaemia in the involved tissues, resulting in impaired resistance to infection. It should also be remembered that many chemotherapeutic agents reduce the white blood cell count drastically and this also reduces resistance to infection of the dental tissues.

Regardless of the treatment, survival is heavily dependent on the stage of the disease at time of treatment (Figs. 3.6 and 3.7). One of the reasons why lip cancers have a higher survival rate than intraoral cancers is that the vast majority of lip cancers are treated when still small, which is not the case with intraoral lesions.

Current knowledge is not sufficient for measures to be proposed for the prevention of oral cancer, but certainly the prevention of much suffering and disfigurement, especially in the elderly, can be achieved by astute and observant clinicians.

ORAL CANDIDIASIS

The yeast-like fungus *Candida albicans* is present in the oral flora of 50% of normal mouths, but it is also the most common cause of mucosal infections. When the yeast produces hyphae that

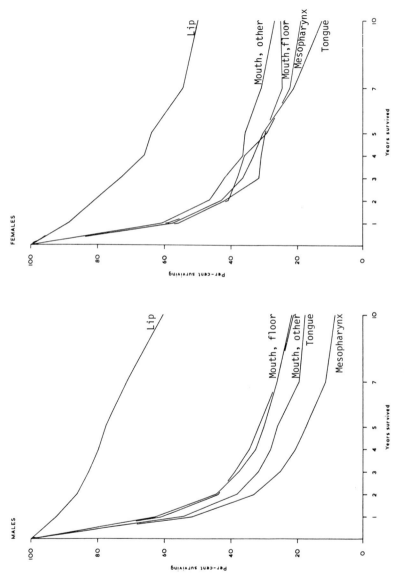

Fig 3.6 *Survival of patients with intraoral cancer of various sites.*

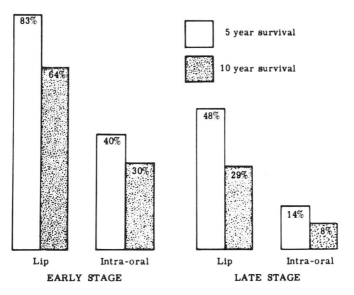

Fig 3.7   *Summary of 5- and 10-year survival rates of early and late stage lip and intraoral cancers.*

invade epithelial cells many different clinical conditions may ensue (Cawson 1984). These include:

acute pseudomembranous candidiasis – thrush
acute atrophic candidiasis – antibiotic sore mouth
chronic atrophic candidiasis – denture-associated stomatitis
chronic hyperplastic candidiasis – candidal leukoplakia
angular cheilitis
median rhomboid glossitis
mucocutaneous candidiasis syndromes (rare and normally
    appearing in childhood)

It is convenient to consider these manifestations individually but it should be understood that they may overlap and many clinical and aetiological features may be present in the same patient.

Aetiological considerations

Some patients who are otherwise in good health and in whom no underlying factor can be found are susceptible to recurrent or persistent candidal infections. Many patients, however, have

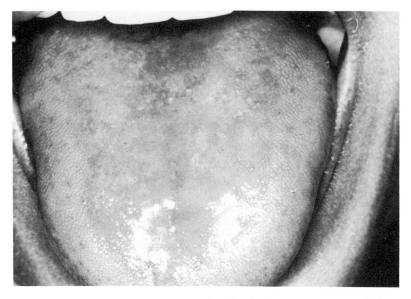

Fig 3.8   *Smooth tongue with superimposed candidal infection in a patient with chronic iron deficiency.*

local or systemic problems that increase their susceptibility. These include:

antibiotic treatment – particularly broad-spectrum antibiotics such as the tetracyclines

immunosuppressive treatment – drugs to prevent transplant rejection or reduce autoimmunity, anticancer chemotherapy, corticosteroids

immune defects – congenital or acquired as a result of disease

iron deficiency (Fig. 3.8) – particularly in cases resistant to treatment (Rennie et al. 1984)

Thrush

This is the best known, though not the most common, form of candidal infection. It is an acute infection characterised by white or cream-coloured plaques that form on the surface of the oral mucosa. The plaques are curd-like in consistency and easily scraped off with a spatula or tongue depressor leaving a red, weeping mucosal surface (Fig. 3.9). The diagnosis is easily confirmed by a direct smear of the plaque material. Masses of strongly Gram-positive hyphae are seen, mixed with desquamated epithelial cells.

Treatment of thrush (as in all candidal infections) involves the elimination of any underlying cause, as well as antifungal therapy. Thrush responds to the topical use of nystatin (500 000 units) lozenges, which are allowed to dissolve in the mouth four times daily. Alternative topical medications include amphotericin B, clotrimazole and miconazole. Effective systemic treatment can be accomplished with ketaconazole (one 200mg tablet daily). This is more convenient for the patient and is particularly helpful in cases where there is a concurrent candidal vulvovaginitis.

Antibiotic sore mouth

This is another acute form of candidal infection. It follows antibiotic therapy, either topically in the form of lozenges or mouth rinses, or from prolonged systemic use of high doses of broad-spectrum antibiotics such as tetracycline. The oral mucosa may

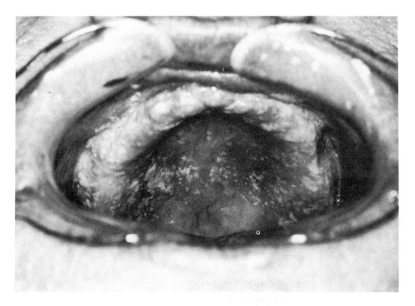

Fig 3.9   *Acute pseudomembranous candidiasis (thrush) in an immunosuppressed elderly patient.*

develop lesions similar to thrush but more frequently the tissues become fiery red and painful and there may be some oedema. Angular cheilitis is a common accompanying feature. The problem will usually resolve with cessation of the antibiotic treatment, but antifungal therapy will hasten recovery.

Denture-associated stomatitis

Denture-associated candidiasis is by far the most common type of oral candidal infection. The characteristic appearance is that of a red mucosa which corresponds exactly to the area covered by a full upper denture. The condition seldom causes any discomfort and hence the term 'denture sore mouth' is not accurate. The problem is more prevalent with acrylic dentures and for years was assumed to be of allergic origin despite the fact that no correctly skin-tested case has ever been proven. Acrylic, because of its fine porosity, allows attachment and colonisation by the fungus (Fig. 3.10). The stability and peripheral seal of an upper denture provides the ideal environment for the fungus to flourish in the absence of normal salivary flow. Accompanying angular

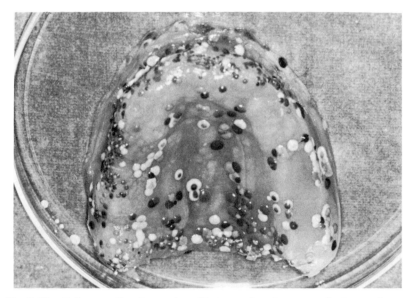

Fig 3.10   *Culture medium impression of fitting surface of upper acrylic denture from a patient with denture-associated stomatitis showing colonies of* Candida albicans.

cheilitis is common, and this is often the patient's original complaint. Management is difficult because disinfecting the denture as well as the mucosal surface is essential. In order to expose the infected tissue to topical antifungal agents, the denture must be left out as much as possible and definitely at night. The denture must be kept scrupulously clean and frequently exposed to a denture cleanser containing a 1% solution of sodium hypochlorite. Many patients of course are not prepared to be seen in public without their dentures and a possible compromise would be to combine the use of nystatin lozenges or systemic ketoconazole with the application of amphotericin B cream to the fitting surface of the denture.

Chronic hyperplastic candidiasis

This is the least common of the oral candidoses but may have very serious implications for the patient. The lesions of chronic candidiasis are true leukoplakias in that they are white lesions which cannot be easily rubbed off. The lesions may be smooth or nodular white plaques or, as is frequently the case, a speckled type of leukoplakia in which there are red and white areas. The diagnosis can only be made by biopsy and it is important for the pathologist to determine the degree of dysplasia, if any, in these lesions. In the past it has been assumed, despite the lack of any supporting evidence, that candidal hyphae were simply superimposed on epithelium which already showed some abnormality such as hyperplasia or dysplasia. Recently (Cawson and Binnie 1980), the simplicity of this assumption has been challenged and it may be that *Candida albicans* in these chronic conditions is not only capable of producing hyperplasia but is possibly involved in the transformation to neoplasia.

Candidal leukoplakias are persistent lesions and, although they may respond partly to antifungal therapy, this is very seldom curative. After two weeks of medication the lesion may have reduced in area and thickness, but surgical excision is then recommended. Although candidal leukoplakias can occur anywhere on the oral mucosa, by far the most common site is the buccal mucosa, particularly near the commissure, followed by the tongue. There is some association between smoking and candidal leukoplakia and, in patients who continue to smoke, many cases either fail to respond to treatment or tend to recur.

Angular cheilitis

Inflammation at the corners of the mouth is a relatively common problem in elderly patients, many of whom, of course, wear full upper and lower dentures. It is important to realise that age changes in the skin and the decreased vertical dimension which produce sagging and obvious folds at the corners of the mouth in the elderly are not responsible for angular cheilitis. This is an infection, most often due to *Candida albicans*, though pathogenic bacteria can be isolated in some cases. It can be associated with any of the types of intraoral candidal infection and indeed is the only sign which is common to all. It is also frequently associated with iron deficiency. The lesions at the oral commissure vary from reddening of the tissues to deep ulcerations and crusted fissures. The treatment of angular cheilitis is to treat the oral infection; obviously, where there is also staphylococcal involvement, the appropriate antibiotic in addition to the anti-fungal drugs must be prescribed. Finally, if there is obvious reduction in the vertical dimension, this should be corrected for prosthetic reasons. This will also reduce the depth of skin folds and thus decrease the seepage of infected saliva into the commissural tissues.

Median rhomboid glossitis

This lesion occurs in the midline of the dorsum of the tongue just anterior to the circumvallate papillae. It is a smooth, red, depapillated or pebbly area with distinctive margins and there may occasionally be white flecks on the surface. In the past the lesion was considered to be a developmental defect due to persistence or lack of submersion of the tuberculum impar. This was obviously a simplistic explanation since a developmental lesion would be obvious from birth. In fact the condition is exceedingly rare in the younger age groups and it has been realised in the last few years that this is another form of localised candidal infection. It may be that this area is particularly prone to infection because of an embryological difference in the tissues in this area. The most important thing about median rhomboid glossitis is to recognise it for what it is. Because of various clinical and histological features, some of these lesions have been mistakenly treated as cancer. This is in fact one of the areas of the mouth in which squamous cell carcinoma is least likely to develop.

In addition to the superficial infections discussed here, *Candida albicans* can also cause systemic infections. These, though uncommon, are severe and often fatal. They are particularly important because of their frequency as a complication of immunosuppressive or cytotoxic treatment, of cardiac surgery, or of other invasive procedures. It is obviously important, therefore, in the elderly or debilitated patient that local infections be eliminated to avoid systemic spread.

HERPES VIRUS INFECTIONS

The only common viral infections of the head and neck that occur in elderly patients are those caused by the herpes viruses, particularly herpes simplex and varicella–zoster. After infection, these viruses are not destroyed but remain dormant in sensory ganglia throughout the patient's life. In the elderly, the viruses may be reactivated by chronic debility or immunosuppression. Although T lymphocyte numbers remain relatively constant throughout life, many T-cell functions are diminished with age. Herpes infections, which are usually mild and self-limiting in healthy patients, can be life-threatening in the immuno-compromised elderly patient.

Reactivated intraoral herpes simplex infections are characterised by an acute vesicular eruption on masticatory mucosa (hard palate or gingiva). The vesicles rupture, leaving clusters of painful shallow ulcers with erythematous borders. These spread and coalesce (Fig. 3.11). Zoster (shingles) is also characterised by an acute and exquisitely painful vesicular eruption. The lesions of zoster, however, can occur on any intraoral surface, are characteristically unilateral and may be accompanied by vesicles on the overlying skin.

Treatment

Life-threatening herpes virus infections in the immunocompromised patient can be successfully managed with intravenous acyclovir in many instances (Selby et al. 1979). Recurrent intra-oral herpes simplex infections are rarely diagnosed at an early stage and are therefore usually managed palliatively with medications such as tetracycline mouth rinses. If a recurrent herpetic lesion can be identified in its prodromal stage, slight clinical

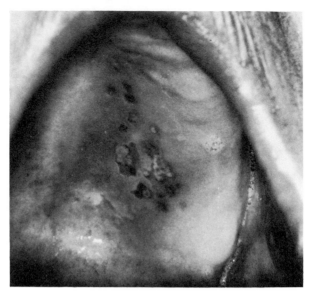

Fig 3.11   *Recurrent intraoral herpes simplex viral infection showing ruptured vesicles on the mucosal surface of the hard palate.*

improvement has been reported using topical 5% acyclovir (Fiddian et al. 1983). Numerous other remedies have been suggested over many years, their multiplicity being an indication of the frequency with which these recurrent lesions occur and the discomfort they cause. A new and most promising development has been the recent discovery by Poswillo and Roberts (1981) that topically-applied carbenoxolone is highly effective for the treatment of acute and recurrent herpetic stomatitis. Subsequently, Partridge and Poswillo (1984) have demonstrated similarly encouraging results for cases of herpes labialis and herpes zoster. While carbenoxolone is most active against HSV1 infections its analogue, cicloxolone, is more effective where HSV2 is the infecting agent (Csonka and Tyrrell 1984). Since the publication of Poswillo's papers there have been many reports from different sources to indicate that treatment with carbenoxolone not only reduces the healing time of labial lesions but that the frequency of subsequent recurrences appears to be progessively reduced; moreover, if treatment can be initiated during the prodromal stage the development of labial lesions can often be aborted.

Herpes zoster is usually managed by a dermatologist, but

guidelines for its treatment and prophylaxis have recently been published (Nicholson 1984).

MUCOCUTANEOUS DISORDERS

These are diseases which are seen by the dermatologist and the dentist. Those of particular concern to the older age group are lichen planus, lupus erythematosus, pemphigus vulgaris, and benign mucous membrane pemphigoid. All produce inflammatory lesions of the oral mucosa but are not associated with any infective microorganism.

Lichen planus

Oral lichen planus is a chronic persistent inflammatory condition of unknown cause. It is seldom found before middle age and is twice as common in women as men. It can affect most areas of the mouth but is most common in the posterior buccal mucosa where it is almost always bilateral although not necessarily symmetrical. Other sites commonly affected are the dorsum and lateral margins of the tongue and gingiva. Less than half of patients with oral lesions ever manifest skin disease. The characteristic skin lesion is a violaceous papule which is intensely itchy and most frequently affects the inside of the forearms and wrists, although the disease has been reported in most other skin sites. In contrast, the oral lesions are symptomless and often discovered incidentally during routine dental examination.

Oral lichen planus can produce many different types of mucosal lesion and this has lead to subclassifications (e.g. hypertrophic, atrophic, erosive, bullous and ulcerative). It is accepted now by most clinicians that subclassification is pointless other than for descriptive purposes since many of these appearances can either be seen in the same patient at any one time or the disease itself will go through changing patterns with time.

The classical description of oral lichen planus is that of a bilateral lace-like or circinate pattern of white lines (the striae of Wickham) on both buccal mucosae (Fig. 3.12). Similar lesions may be seen on the tongue but usually in this site the dorsum has a homogeneous white or silvery sheen generally with some degree of depapillation. Even in these homogeneous lesions the white lacy pattern may be seen at the periphery, particularly if

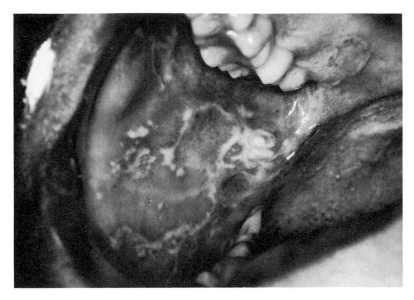

Fig 3.12 *Lichen planus. The characteristic white striae of Wickham were bilaterally present on the buccal mucosa.*

the tongue is stretched. These hypertrophic lesions are normally symptomless and, if questioned, the patient may only be aware of some roughness of the cheeks. Symptoms occur when the epithelium becomes thin and the area is described as erosive or atrophic (which are not strictly accurate descriptions). The mucosa takes on an erythematous appearance and patients complain of a burning sensation. This of course tends to be exacerbated in areas where there is additional mild trauma and probably explains why the site of most frequent complaint is the posterior buccal mucosa, where the tissues are in contact with the buccal surfaces of the molar teeth. With increasing inflammation the surface epithelium may be shed, leading to shallow ulceration or peeling of the surface.

Frank ulceration in lichen planus, particularly in the dorsum of the tongue, has a characteristic appearance. The ulcers tend to be large (greater than 1.5cm in diameter), have well defined margins with no erythema and are covered by an exceedingly tough fibrinous surface. They are classically described as indolent in that there is very little change over periods of weeks. They appear to be neither healing nor getting worse. Although looking disturbing to the clinician, they produce surprisingly little discomfort compared with erosive areas.

Gingival lesions may be localised and patchy, or may affect the whole of the attached gingiva and alveolar mucosa. The interdental papillae are often spared. A striate appearance is rare and most often the whole of gingival mucosa appears as a fiery red, smooth oedematous area traditionally described as 'desquamative gingivitis'.

Management

If oral lichen planus is symptomless, it needs no treatment. If there is any doubt about the diagnosis, for instance whether or not the lesions constitute a speckled leukoplakia, then biopsy is essential. Oral lichen planus is not curable and it is probable that, although the appearance and symptoms may wax and wane, the condition may be present in some form for the rest of the patient's life. Significant improvement can normally be achieved with corticosteroids. If the lesions are particularly severe and widespread, initial management may require systemic therapy with 20–25mg of prednisolone daily. Improvement should be seen within four or five days and maintenance or further improvement may be achieved with topical application. In the United Kingdom the most effective topical corticosteroid is betamethasone valerate (0.1mg) pellets. The pellet is allowed to dissolve as close as possible to the source of discomfort and up to four pellets a day can be rotated around different troublesome areas of the mouth. Gingival symptoms may be relieved with triamcinolone (in Orabase) applied directly to the tissues. It is important to realise however that, since lichen planus is an inflammatory condition, any contributing local irritation will make the symptoms worse. It is therefore necessary in the case of gingival lesions that dental plaque be eliminated in order to avoid contributing to the problem.

Another factor to consider in this condition is the psychological make-up of the patient. Lichen planus is usually only seen in patients with an anxious, conscientious type of personality. Furthermore, the lesions are likely to flare up if patients are under extra emotional stress (or for instance, stop smoking) and a course of an anxiolytic agent (e.g. diazepam) in mild doses for a trial period may prove useful not only in reducing the symptoms but also improving the mucosal condition.

Lupus erythematosus

Lupus erythematosus only rarely affects the oral mucosa and is mentioned here because the lesions often bear a striking resemblance both clinically and histologically to lichen planus. A more complete review is provided by Pindborg (1980).

Lupus erythematosus is a broad spectrum of diseases and is traditionally classified into a chronic discoid type and an acute systemic type, but there is frequent overlap between the two. The condition, especially the systemic type, is much more common in females than males. Oral lesions seldom occur in the absence of skin involvement and the patient may well have the classical violaceous butterfly-shaped rash over the bridge of the nose and malar areas or discoid plaques or scars in other areas of the face.

The oral lesions are very variable in appearance, particularly in systemic lupus erythematosus (SLE), but usually appear as multiple discrete erythematous plaques, possibly with some radiating white lines which may resemble the striae of Wickham. The centre of the plaque may ulcerate and the dentist should be suspicious of a patient with multiple painful 'craggy' ulcers with a white radiating halo.

Lupus erythematosus comprises a group of immunological disorders and the patient should be referred to a physician to assess systemic involvement.

Pemphigus vulgaris

Pemphigus vulgaris is a rare but invariably fatal disease if untreated. It is characterised by the formation of vesicles and bullae on the skin and mucous membranes and, in the majority of cases, the first manifestations may be in the mouth. It seldom occurs before middle age and is more common in Ashkenazi Jews than in any other racial group.

Vesicles occur within the epithelium because of loss of cohesion between the cells of the prickle-cell layer (acantholysis). There is an immunological basis for this; a raised titre of antibodies to the intercellular substance of the epithelium (as well as the C3 component of complement) can be demonstrated by immunofluorescence to be deposited between the epithelial cells. These antibodies are tissue-specific and react only to intercellular material of stratified squamous epithelium. Any doubts arising about the diagnosis from routine histological material can be resolved by using immunofluorescent techniques.

When the epithelial cells lose their attachment they become rounded in shape and the cytoplasm contracts. These acantholytic cells are contained in the vesicular fluid and can be seen in microscopic examination of a smear of affected tissue.

The vesicles of pemphigus, because they are covered by thin epithelium, are fragile and they are seldom seen intact within the mouth. The most common appearance is that of several irregular erosions that are tender and often have a haemorrhagic appearance. The characteristic clinical sign in pemphigus is the production of a vesicular bulla by gentle stroking of the skin (Nikolsky's sign). The same phenomenon occurs with stroking of the oral mucosa but is not diagnostic since the effect can also be produced in pemphigoid (see below). Because of the fragility of the epithelium, lesions are likely to develop with minor trauma. The gingivae are commonly affected and pemphigus vulgaris is another cause of desquamative gingivitis.

The disease is variable in its rate of progress but eventually the lesions spread over the surface of the body, loss of fluid and electrolytes from the raw areas becomes severe, and the lesions readily become infected. It is obviously important that the diagnosis be confirmed as soon as possible, especially since immunosuppressive therapy has changed the prognosis drastically. A combination of corticosteroids with newer agents such as azathioprine, usually on alternating days, has produced the most effective results with low enough doses to avoid severe side-effects. Treatment will usually be lifelong but most patients with proper control can assume a normal life expectancy.

Benign mucous membrane (cicatricial) pemphigoid

As the name suggests this is a pemphigus-like condition in that it is a chronic disease causing vesiculobullous lesions and painful erosions. It is more common than pemphigus vulgaris but is not life-threatening.

This is again an immunologically-mediated disease, and the same antibody and complement factors can be demonstrated as in pemphigus vulgaris. However, the problem in pemphigoid occurs at the basement membrane and results in separation of the whole thickness of epithelium from the underlying connective tissues. There is no acantholysis.

Women are affected more often than men and are usually elderly. The mucous membrane of the mouth is affected more frequently, and usually earlier, than other mucosal surfaces. Bullae are produced with minor trauma and can often be seen intact. When they rupture, raw areas are left which are well demarcated from the surrounding mucosa. These erosions may persist for weeks and then heal slowly with scarring. The gingivae are frequently involved and pemphigoid is the second most common cause (after lichen planus) of desquamative gingivitis (Fig. 3.13).

Biopsy is essential for confirmation of the diagnosis, but this may be difficult to achieve because the epithelium often slides away in front of the cutting edge of the scalpel. A healthy oral mucosa can often be attained with the use of topical cortico-steroids such as prednisolone pellets but it is important that the patient be referred for an ophthalmic consultation. Because the lesions and mucosal surfaces heal with scarring, corneal involvement can result in impaired sight or even blindness.

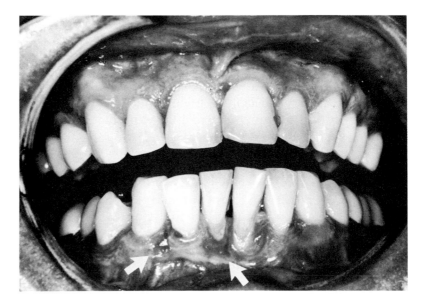

Fig 3.13   *Benign mucous membrane pemphigoid. Ruptured bulla (between arrows) produces 'desquamative gingivitis'.*

DRUG REACTIONS

Most elderly people have at least one chronic illness for which they are receiving medication. In one study, 87% of elderly patients took drugs regularly and a third took three or four drugs daily (Law and Chalmers 1976). Not only do the elderly commonly take drugs, but they are much more likely to have adverse reactions to those drugs than are younger patients (Vestal 1978). Metabolic causes underlying this vulnerability are discussed in Chapter 4.

The oral manifestations of drug reactions are protean, but include (either singly or in combination) stomatitis, necrosis, opportunistic infection, bleeding, gingival hyperplasia, pigmentation, altered salivary function and altered taste. Unfortunately, these clinical changes are not pathognomonic for drug reactions, because each of them can result from conditions unrelated to medication. Most drug-induced oral changes are reversible and alteration or elimination of the drug, in consultation with the prescriber, often results in resolution of the clinical problem.

Although more extensive reviews of drug reactions have been published (Wright 1984), a brief description of the clinical manifestations of drug reactions will be presented. Individual drugs associated with the various reactions are listed in Table 3.1.

Stomatitis

Many drugs are capable of causing intraoral inflammation or stomatitis. Clinically this results in erythema which is often painful. The stomatitis can either be nonspecific or else have specifically distinguishing features to allow subclassification as allergic stomatitis, lichenoid drug reactions, lupus-like drug reactions, or erythema multiforme.

The most common group of drugs inducing nonspecific stomatitis is the antineoplastic or chemotherapeutic drugs used to treat various malignancies. Other drugs reported to cause stomatitis include phenylbutazone, gold, indomethacin and methyldopa.

Allergic stomatitis

The mechanism that produces the stomatitis in some patients is a hypersensitivity or allergic reaction. This can occur from topical

Table 3.1

Drug reactions

Lichenoid reaction

Chloroquine	Methyldopa	Spironolactone
Chlorpropamide	Para-amino salicylic	Streptomycin
Dapsone	acid	Tetracycline
Frusemide	Penicillamine	Thiazides
Gold	Phenothiazines	Tolbutamide
Hydroxychloroquine	Propranolol	Triprolidine
Mercury	Quinidine	

Lupus-like reaction

Gold	Methyldopa	Procainamide
Griseofulvin	Penicillin	Streptomycin
Hydralazine	Phenytoin	Troxidone
Isoniazid	Primidone	

Erythema multiforme

Antimalarials	Clindamycin	Phenytoin
Barbiturates	Codeine	Salicylates
Busulphan	Penicillin	Sulfonamides
Carbamazepine	Phenylbutazone	Tetracyclines
Chlorpropamide		

Necrosis

Silver nitrate	Peroxide	Pancreatic extracts
Phenols	Sodium perborate	Potassium chloride
Acids or alkalis	Gentian violet	

Neutropenia/agranulocytosis

Aminopyrines	Chloramphenicol	Phenylbutazone
Azathioprine	Chlorpromazine	Phenytoin
Barbiturates	Gold salts	Pyribenzamine
Bismuth	Indomethacin	Quinine
Cephalothin	Phenacetin	Sulfonamides
Chemotherapeutic	Phenindione	Tolbutamide
agents	Phenothiazines	Troxidone

Thrombocytopenia

Allopurinol	Cimetidine	Mercurial diuretics
Amphotericin B	Digitalis	Methyldopa
Carbamazepine	Digoxin	Morphine
Cephalosporins	Erythromycin	Paracetamol
Chemotherapeutic	Gold	Penicillin
agents	Heparin	Pethidine
Chloramphenicol	Levamisole	Phenacetin
Codeine	Meprobamate	Phenylbutazone

Thrombocytopenia cont.

Phenytoin	Streptomycin	Tetracycline
Quinidine	Sulfonamide	Tolbutamide
Quinine	Thiazide diuretics	

Soft-tissue pigmentation

Antimalarial drugs	Busulphan	Phenolphthalein
High dose ACTH	Mercurial diuretics	Phenothiazines
Adriamycin	Oral contraceptives	Silver compounds

Xerostomia

Amphetamines	Antispasmodics	Hypnotics
Anticholinergics	Appetite suppressants	Muscle relaxants
(Atropine)	Decongestants	Narcotics
Anti-Parkinsonians	Diuretics	Minor and major
Anticonvulsants	Hypotensives	tranquillisers
Antihistamines	(ganglionic blockers)	Sympathomimetics
Antidepressants		
(tricyclic)		

Salivary gland pain and/or swelling

Bretylium	Isoproterenol	Sulfonamides
Clonidine	Methyldopa	Tri-iodothyronine
Diatrizoate	Oxyphenbutazone	Vinblastine
Guanethidine	Phenothiazines	Vincristine
Insulin	Phenylbutazone	Warfarin sodium
Iodides	Potassium chlorate	

Taste alteration

Amphetamines	Gold	Lithium carbonate
Carbimazole	Griseofulvin	Metronidazole
Clofibrate	Levodopa	Penicillamine
Dimethyl sulphoxide	Lincomycin	Tranquillisers
Ethionamide		

contact with the allergen (stomatitis venenata) or from systemic administration (stomatitis medicamentosa). Both reactions are histamine mediated and result from the reaction of the allergen with IgE antibody on the surface of mast cells. This reaction results in the release of histamine. Both allergic and hypersensitivity reactions require prior sensitisation and occur immediately after allergenic challenge. Stomatitis venenata involves only the tissue contacting the allergen, while stomatitis medicamentosa, being a systemic reaction, tends to be symmetrical, involves larger areas, and is often accompanied by urticaria.

Allergic reactions often begin with a tingling or burning sensation, followed by vesiculation and stomatitis. Eversole (1979) has published a comprehensive review of oral allergies and discusses some of the more common allergens, which include topical medications, antibiotics, additives in mouth rinses and dentifrices, flavouring agents, nickel and soap.

Lichenoid drug reactions

A reaction clinically indistinguishable from lichen planus can follow the administration of drugs. The reaction is usually erosive and may involve the lips, floor of the mouth, and palate, which are areas not commonly affected by lichen planus.

Lupus erythematosus-like drug reactions

Patients taking certain medications can experience a reaction with features similar to systemic lupus erythematosus. These patients develop fever, adenopathy, pleuropulmonary, cardiac and joint symptoms as well as intraoral erythema and ulceration.

Erythema multiforme

Erythema multiforme is an acute immune-mediated mucocutaneous reaction which can be triggered by medication. The skin lesions are highly variable but often involve the palms of the hands and soles of the feet and may appear as a 'target' or 'bull's-eye'. The oral manifestation is characterised by a symmetrical, vesiculobullous stomatitis. Lip involvement resulting in haemorrhagic crusting is highly characteristic. Although classically considered a dermatological condition, erythema multiforme can occur in the absence of skin manifestations (Lozada and Silverman 1978).

Necrosis

There are numerous chemicals that, if placed in contact with the mucosa, will cause necrosis of the surface epithelium. Depending on the duration and severity of the tissue damage, ulceration may result. The classic example is the 'aspirin burn'.

Opportunistic infection

The most common opportunistic infection seen in dental practice is candidiasis, and one of the common predisposing factors is the administration of such drugs as antibiotics, steroids (including aerosol sprays), chemotherapeutic agents and immunosuppressive drugs. With the exception of the chronic hyperplastic type, any of the other clinical types of candidiasis can be drug-induced, and these may be accompanied by angular cheilitis (see p. 58).

Other oral opportunistic infections occur because of drug-induced bone-marrow suppression. Some drugs are capable of destroying neutrophils (neutropenia or agranulocytosis) and/or lymphocytes (immunosuppression). The resulting infections can be bacterial, viral or fungal, and it is important to remember that the mouth is one of the most common sites for infection in compromised hosts.

The classic oral manifestation of agranulocytosis is ragged, poorly-healing ulcerations. Common oral infections such as periodontitis, which are to some extent held in check by host responses, will progress rapidly if those responses are reduced or eliminated.

Haemorrhage

Bleeding can occur in patients on medications and usually results from the suppression of the production of platelets or thrombocytes (thrombocytopenia). Thrombocytopenia results in petechiae or ecchymoses of the skin and mucous membranes. Frank bleeding, often from the gingiva, is seen.

Gingival hyperplasia

Diffuse gingival enlargement as a side-effect of phenytoin for the treatment of seizures is well known. The severity of the hyperplasia is related to the degree of local irritation and inadequacy of oral hygiene. The hyperplasia can be controlled or prevented in some patients by meticulous attention to oral hygiene.

Other drugs which can induce a similar hyperplasia include primidone, cyclosporin (Wysocki et al. 1983) and nifedipine (Lederman et al. 1984).

Pigmentation

A linear pigmentation can be seen along the marginal gingiva in patients who have ingested heavy metals such as lead, mercury, bismuth and cis platinum.

The teeth can be discoloured in patients taking tetracycline, liquid iron, chlorhexidine and large quantities of fluoride; tetracycline and excessive fluoride are particularly to be avoided during tooth development.

Multiple areas of soft-tissue pigmentation can be seen in patients taking medication.

Altered salivary function

Xerostomia

The most common drug-induced alteration of salivary gland function is xerostomia, and there are over 250 drugs which have been identified as capable of causing this side-effect (Bahn 1972). This is a particularly relevant problem for the elderly, most of whom are taking medication (see p. 116).

Salivary gland pain and/or swelling

Some drugs occasionally cause pain or swelling of the salivary glands, usually the parotids.

Taste alteration

Patients on medication may report an alteration of sense of taste.

XEROSTOMIA

Xerostomia, or dry mouth, is an ever increasing problem for the elderly. It may well be part of the normal effects of ageing. With age, there is continued loss of parasympathetic tone as well as fatty and fibrous infiltration of the parenchyma of the major salivary glands (Waterhouse et al. 1973). Also, as discussed in Chapter 2, the volume of acinar tissue diminishes progressively. Although decreased salivation in the elderly as a totally age-related phenomenon has recently been challenged (Mandel

1984), the fact remains that clinically a dry, sore mouth is a common complaint of the elderly, and an understanding of its causes and effects is imperative for those providing dental care for these patients.

Aetiology

Xerostomia is not a disease, but a sign or symptom of some underlying pathophysiological process. The causes of xerostomia are numerous and varied, but Mason and Chisholm (1975) have proposed a workable classification (Table 3.2).

One of the most common causes of xerostomia in the elderly is a side-effect of medication (Table 3.1). Emotional disturbances such as depression or anxiety are commonly seen in this age group and these disturbances and/or their treatment often result in a dry mouth. The most common chronic illness affecting old

Table 3.2

Causes of xerostomia

1. Factors affecting the salivary centre
   a. Emotional – fear, excitement, anxiety
   b. Neuroses – depression
   c. Organic disease of the central nervous system (CNS) – tumours
   d. Drugs
2. Factors affecting autonomic output
   a. CNS alterations – inflammation, tumours, surgery, trauma
   b. Drugs
3. Factors affecting salivary gland function
   a. Aplasia
   b. Obstruction and trauma
   c. Sjögren's syndrome
   d. Infection
   e. Irradiation
4. Factors affecting fluid or electrolyte balance
   a. Dehydration
   b. Diabetes mellitus and insipidus
   c. Heart and kidney failure
   d. Oedema
   e. Anaemia
5. Local factors
   a. Mouth breathing
   b. Excessive smoking

Adapted from Mason and Chisholm (1975)

people is cardiovascular disease, and numerous patients will be taking diuretics or antihypertensives, many of which cause xerostomia. It is important to remember that many of the drugs which cause xerostomia can be purchased without a prescription, and the elderly tend to self-prescribe over-the-counter medications much more commonly than the general adult population (Guttmann 1977). Taking a drug history from such patients can be complicated by the fact that medications may be prescribed by more than one clinician and, in addition, many do not know what drugs they are taking or why.

Other causes of xerostomia are those primary conditions of the glands which affect function. Because most secretion comes from the parotid and submaxillary glands, it is rare for a single tumour to reduce salivary flow significantly. The same is true for inflammatory or obstructive disorders of single glands, with the notable exception of some of the granulomatous diseases. Sarcoidosis has a distinct tendency to involve multiple salivary glands and can result in xerostomia. Sarcoid of the parotids which causes facial paralysis and eye involvement (uveitis) is known as Heerfordt's syndrome.

Sjögren's syndrome

Sjögren's syndrome is a major cause of xerostomia in some series (Spielman et al. 1981). Sjögren's syndrome (sicca syndrome) is an autoimmune disease of exocrine glands and primarily affects the salivary and lacrimal glands. It is seen most often in middle-aged to elderly females and is characterised by progressive infiltration of the glands with lymphoid tissue which results in parenchymal destruction. Sjögren's syndrome occurs alone as a limited disease (primary), or in conjunction with other auto-immune diseases (secondary), most commonly with rheumatoid arthritis (Snider 1975).

Most patients with Sjögren's syndrome will experience unilateral or bilateral intermittent swelling of their parotid glands. The swelling is firm and painless, a feature which distinguishes it from inflammatory enlargement. The absence of swelling, however, does not preclude the diagnosis because many patients will not have demonstrable swelling at the time of examination. As exocrine gland function diminishes, patients complain of a dry, sore mouth and a gritty feeling in their eyes.

The diagnosis of Sjögren's syndrome has historically been

made when two out of three of the classic triad are present. These include xerostomia, xerophthalmia and an autoimmune rheumatic disorder. Labial salivary gland biopsy has been advocated as an adjunct to diagnosis because of the frequent occurrence of lymphocytic infiltrates in the glands of Sjögren's patients (Tarpley et al. 1974). However, similar infiltrates can be seen in the labial salivary glands of patients with autoimmune disorders without Sjögren's syndrome (Friedman et al. 1979) and have even been documented in patients with xerostomia only (Spielman et al. 1982). Sialochemistry has demonstrated an increase in salivary sodium, potassium and IgA in Sjögren patients (Spielman et al. 1982). Although numerous serological parameters are altered, most patients have specific autoantibodies against salivary ductal epithelium.

Radiation therapy is a well-known cause of xerostomia. The decrease in salivation shows a linear correlation with the accumulated radiation dosage (Mira et al. 1982) and most patients will experience irreversible xerostomia after about 4 000 rads (40Gy).

More rarely, xerostomia results from alteration of autonomic output in the central nervous system or as a manifestation of a systemic condition. Chronic anxiety states and depression are common causes, as well as those conditions resulting in fluid depletion.

Effects of xerostomia

Xerostomia often results in predictable signs and symptoms as a result of the loss of normal salivary functions. Patients have trouble eating and talking as their dry mucosa adheres to itself. They complain of soreness or burning as a result of the physical irritation due to lack of lubrication. This symptom is often worsened with superimposed candidiasis, and patients may exhibit angular cheilitis (Fig. 3.14a). Many elderly subjects wear removable prostheses and these are particularly irritating to the underlying mucosa in the absence of the normal mucous barrier between the denture and tissues. Some patients experience a loss of taste sense which decreases appetite. The symptoms of xerostomia are sometimes sufficiently disabling to cause anxiety and depression, which further worsens the xerostomia.

Examination of the patient often reveals a dry mouth with decreased quantities of saliva although xerostomia is admittedly a subjective diagnosis. The saliva is often viscous and frothy. As

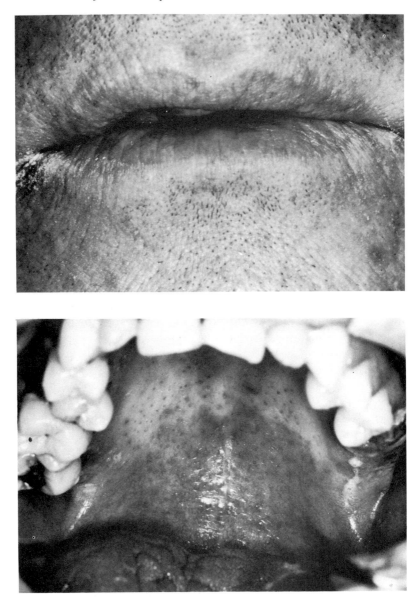

Fig 3.14   *This 52-year-old male was referred for evaluation of uncontrollable caries. He had a sore, dry mouth due primarily to multiple medications prescribed for the control of chronic anxiety and depression. His mucosa was dry and erythematous. Physical irritation with superimposed candidiasis resulted in (a) angular cheilitis and (b) stomatitis.*

a result of the physical irritation and/or candidiasis, the mucosa appears red and atrophic (Fig. 3.14b). Severe cases may show fissuring and ulceration. With decreased salivation, plaque accumulates and the tongue may become coated. Some patients experience halitosis.

It is now known that the increased incidence of dental caries in irradiated patients is due entirely to the effects of xerostomia. All patients with prolonged xerostomia are at an increased risk for caries development and this is characteristically root-surface caries (Jordan and Summer 1973).

Management

Management of the dry mouth must begin with an assessment of the underlying cause. If a specific aetiologic factor (e.g. diabetes) can be identified, the first step would obviously entail treating the general condition and not the xerostomia.

A drug history is mandatory in evaluating dry-mouth patients, particularly in the elderly, and should ascertain over-the-counter medications. If an offending drug can be identified, consultation with the prescriber can determine whether the drug can be eliminated or changed. For instance, the anticholinergic effect of a tricyclic antidepressant results in significant mucosal drying; switching to one of the newer tetracyclic compounds will often relieve oral symptoms without compromising therapeutic efficacy. In addition, giving some drugs more frequently during the day in smaller doses can reduce the xerostomia.

If a cause cannot be identified or if a patient has intrinsically lost the ability to produce saliva (e.g. Sjögren's syndrome, radiation), then management is directed towards reducing the effects of the xerostomia, and making the patient more comfortable.

Patients should be instructed to avoid dry foods as well as spicy or acidic foods which are irritating to an already inflamed mucosa. Alcohol and smoking will further dry the mucosa. It is important that patients take plenty of fluids and maintain good hydration but they must avoid caffeinated beverages because of the diuretic properties of caffeine.

Salivary stimulants provide relief for some patients. Lemon flavouring is one of the best salivary stimulants but chewing gum or other flavoured sugar-free candies also provide salivary stimulation. Under no circumstance should sugar-containing mints or candies be prescribed for prolonged periods of time because of the caries susceptibility of xerostomic patients. Spielman and associates (1981) have recommended a mouthwash containing citric acid as a salivary stimulant but, because citric acid is a potent chelator (Newbrun 1981), long-term use could result in erosion of the teeth. On occasion, systemic autonomic stimulation of salivary function with pilocarpine or a cholinesterase inhibitor can be achieved. However, these drugs are not specific for salivary stimulation and side-effects should be expected.

Numerous commercially-available saliva substitutes can be used for replacement therapy, and these provide significant relief. They can be purchased without a prescription and substitutes containing fluoride have proved beneficial. These can be used as often as needed and can also be applied to prostheses.

In dentulous patients with severe xerostomia, topical fluoride applications are recommended and meticulous oral hygiene should be maintained (Beumer et al. 1979). A sucrose-free diet should be encouraged.

This chapter has dealt with those oral mucosal diseases that we feel are most common or of most concern to this age group. Many mucosal problems result from medication and systemic disease. Diligence in medical history-taking and understanding the implications of the various medical problems encountered is, therefore, of particular importance when dealing with elderly patients.

REFERENCES

Axell T., Holmstrup P., Kramer I. R. H., Pindborg J. J., Shear M. (1984). International seminar on oral leukoplakia and associated lesions related to tobacco habits. *Community Dent. Oral Epidemiol.*; **12**: 146–54.

Bahn S. L. (1972). Drug related dental destruction. *Oral Surg.*; **33**: 49–54.

Beumer J., Curtis T., Harrison R. E. (1979). Radiation therapy of the oral cavity: Sequelae and management, Part 2. *Head and Neck Surg.*; **1**: 392–408.

Binnie W. H., Rankin K. V., Mackenzie I. C. (1983). Etiology of oral squamous cell carcinoma. *J. Oral. Path.*; **12**: 11–29.

Cawson R. A. (1984). In *Essentials of Dental Surgery and Pathology*, 4th edn., Chap. 15. New York: Churchill Livingstone.

Cawson R. A., Binnie W. H. (1980). Candida leukoplakia and carcinoma: A possible relationship. In *Oral Premalignancy* (Mackenzie I. C., Dabelsteen E., Squier C. A., eds.) pp. 59–66. Iowa City: University of Iowa Press.

Cooke B. E. D. (1956). Leukoplakia buccalis and oral epithelial naevi. Clinical and histological study. *Br. J. Dermatol.*; **68**: 151–74.

Csonka G. W., Tyrrell D. A. J. (1984). Treatment of herpes genitalis with carbenoxolone and cicloxalone creams. *Br. J. Ven. Dis.*; **60**: 178–81.

Doll R., Hill A. B. (1964). Mortality in relation to smoking: ten years' observation of British doctors. *Br. Med. J.*; **1**: 1399–410; 1460–7.

Eversole L. R. (1979). Allergic stomatitides. *J. Oral Med.*; **34**: 93–102.

Fiddian A. P., Yeo J. M., Stubbings R. et al. (1983). Successful treatment of herpes labialis with topical acyclovir. *Br. Med. J.*; **286**: 1699–701.

Fischman S. L., Martinez I. (1977). Oral cancer in Puerto Rico. *J. Surg. Oncol.*; **9**: 163–9.

Friedman H., Kilmar V., Galletta V. P. et al. (1979). Lip biopsy in connective tissue diseases. A review and study of seventy cases. *Oral Surg.*; **47**: 256–62.

Guttmann D. (1977). Patterns of legal drug use by older Americans. *Addict. Dis.*; **3**: 337–56.

Jordan H. V., Summer D. L. (1973). Root surface caries: Review of the literature and significance of the problem. *J. Periodontol.*; **44**: 158–62.

Joynson D. H., Walker D. M., Jacobs A., Dolby A. E. (1972). Defect of cell-mediated immunity in patients with iron-deficiency anaemia. *Lancet*; ii: 1058–9.

Kelly A. B. (1919). Spasm at the entrance of the esophagus. *J. Laryngol.*; **34**: 285–9.

Kramer I. R. H., El-Labban N., Lee K. W. (1978). The clinical features and risk of malignant transformation in sublingual keratosis. *Br. Dent. J.*; **144**: 171–80.

Law R., Chalmers C. (1976). Medicines and elderly people: A general practice survey. *Br. Med. J.*; **1**: 565–8.

Lederman D., Lumerman H., Reuben S. et al. (1984). Gingival hyperplasia associated with nifedipine therapy. *Oral Surg.*; **57**: 620–2.

Levin M. L., Goldstein H., Gerhardt P. R. (1950). Cancer and tobacco smoking. *J.A.M.A.*; **143**: 336–8.

Lozada F., Silverman S. (1978). Erythema multiforme. Clinical characteristics and natural history in 50 patients. *Oral Surg.*; **46**: 628–36.

Mahboubi E. (1977). The epidemiology of oral cavity, pharyngeal and esophageal cancer outside of North America and Western Europe. *Cancer*; **40**: 1879–86.

Mandel I. D. (1984). Oral defenses and disease: Salivary gland function. *Gerondontol.*; **3**: 47–54.

Martinez I. (1969). Factors associated with cancer of the oesophagus, mouth and pharynx in Puerto Rico. *J. Natl. Cancer Inst.*; **42**: 1069–94.

Mashberg A. (1978). Erythroplasia: the earliest sign of asymptomatic oral cancer. *J. Am. Dent. Assoc.*; **96**: 615–20.

Mashberg A., Garfinkel L., Harris S. (1981). Alcohol as a primary risk factor in oral squamous carcinoma. *C.A.*; **31**: 146–55.

Mashberg A., Meyers H. (1976). Anatomical site and size of 222 early asymptomatic oral squamous cell carcinomas. *Cancer*; **37**: 2149–57.

Mason D. K., Chisholm D. M. (1975). *Salivary Glands in Health and Disease*. London, W. B. Saunders, Co. p. 120.

Massé L. (1972). Epidemiology of cancer of the oesophagus in Brittany. *Typescript of special lecture in the University of London*.

Mira J. G., Fullerton G. D., Wescott W. B. (1982). Correlation between initial salivary flow rate and radiation dose in the production of xerostomia. *Acta. Radiol. Oncol.*; **21**: 151–4.

Newbrun E. (1981). Xerostomia. *Oral Surg.*; **52**: 262.

Nicholson K. G. (1984). Antiviral agents in clinical practice. Antiviral therapy. Varicella-zoster virus infections, herpes labialis and mucocutaneous herpes, and cytomegalovirus infections. *Lancet*; ii: 677–82.

Panagopoulos A. P. (1959). Bone involvement in maxillofacial cancer. *Am. J. Surg.*; **98**: 898–903.

Partridge Maxine, Poswillo D. E. (1984). Topical carbenoxolone sodium in the management of herpes simplex infection. *Br. J. Oral & Maxillofac. Surg.*; **22**: 138–45.

Paterson D. R. (1919). A clinical type of dysphagia. *J. Laryngol.*; **34**: 289–91.

Pindborg J. J. (1980). Diseases of the skin. In *Oral Manifestations of Systemic Disease* (Jones J. H., Mason D. K., eds.) 1st edn., Chapter 12. London: W. B. Saunders Company Ltd.

Poswillo D. E., Roberts G. J. (1981). Topical carbenoxolone for orofacial herpes simplex infection. *Lancet*; i: 143.

Power, D'Arcy (1918). On cancer of the tongue. The Bradshaw lecture, 1918. *Br. J. Surg.*; **6**: 336–50.

Rawles W. E., Tompkins W. A. F., Figueroa M. E., Melnick J. L. (1968). Herpes virus Type 2: Association with carcinoma of the cervix. *Science*; **161**: 1255–6.

Rennie J. S., MacDonald D. G., Dagg J. H. (1984). Iron and the oral epithelium: a review. *J. R. Soc. Med.*; **77**: 602–7.

Rothman K. J. (1978). The effect of alcohol consumption on risk of cancer of the head and neck. *Laryngoscope Suppl. 8.*; **88**: 51–5.

Rothman K. J., Keller A. Z. (1972). The effect of joint exposure to alcohol and tobacco on risk of cancer of the mouth and pharynx. *J. Chronic Dis.*; **25**: 711–16.

Schwartz D., Lellouch J., Flamant R., Denoix P. F. (1962). Aocoolet cancer. Resultats d'une enquete retrospective. *Rev. Franc. Etud. Clini. Biol.*; **7**: 590–604.

Selby P. J., Jameson B., Watson J. G., et al. (1979). Parenteral acyclovir therapy for herpesvirus infections in man. *Lancet*; ii: 1267–70.

Shillitoe E. J., Greenspan D., Greenspan, J. S., Hansen L. S., Silverman S. Jr. (1982). Neutralising antibody to Herpes simplex virus Type 1 in patients with oral cancer. *Cancer*; **49**: 2315–20.

Smith H. G., Cretien P. B., Henson D. E., Silverman N. A., Alexander J. C. (1976). Viral specific humoral immunity to herpes simplex-induced antigens in patients with squamous carcinoma of the head and neck. *Am. J. Surg.*; **132**: 541–8.

Snider G. L. (1975). Case 28–1975, in case records of the Massachusetts General Hospital. *New Engl. J. Med.*; **293**: 136–44.

Spielman A., Ben-Arych H., Gutman D. et al. (1981). Xerostomia – Diagnosis and Treatment. *Oral Surg.*; **51**: 144–7.

Spielman A., Ben-Aryeh H., Lichtig C. et al. (1982). Correlation between sialochemistry and lip biopsy in Sjögren's syndrome patients. *Int. J. Oral Surg.*; **11**: 326–30.

Tarpley T. M., Anderson L. G., White C. L. (1974). Minor salivary gland involvement in Sjögren's syndrome. *Oral Surg.*; **37**: 64–74.

Trieger N., Ship I, I., Taylor G. W., Weisberger D. (1958). Cirrhosis and other predisposing factors in carcinoma of the tongue. *Cancer*; **11**: 357–62.

Vestal R. E. (1978). Drug use in the elderly: A review of problems and special considerations. *Drugs*; **16**: 358–82.

Waldron C. A. (1970). Oral epithelial tumours. In *Thoma's Oral Pathology* (Gorlin R. J., Goldman H. M., eds.) 6th edn., Chap. 19. St. Louis: C. V. Mosby Co.

Waldron C. A., Shafer W. G. (1975). Leukoplakia revisited: A clinicopathologic study of 3256 oral leukoplakias. *Cancer*; **36**: 1386–92.

Waterhouse J. P., Chisholm D. M., Winter R. B. et al. (1973). Replacement of functional parenchymal cells by fat and connective tissue in human submandibular salivary glands: An age related change. *J. Oral Pathol.*; **2**: 16–27.

Winn D. M., Blot W. J., Shy C. M., Pickle L. W., Toledo A., Fraumen J. F. Jr. (1981). Snuff dipping and oral cancer among women in the southern United States. *New Engl. J. Med.*; **304**: 745–9.

Wright J. M. (1984). Oral manifestations of drug reactions. In *Dental Clinics of North America Symposium of Pharmacology and Therapeutics*. (Gage T., ed.). Philadelphia: W. B. Saunders Co., pp. 529–43.

Wynder E. L., Bross I. J., Feldman R. M. (1957). A study of the etiological factors in cancer of the mouth. *Cancer*; **10**: 1300–23.

Wysocki G. P., Gretzinger H. A., Laupacia A. et al. (1983). Fibrous hyperplasia of the gingiva. A side effect of cyclosporin A therapy. *Oral Surg.*; **55**: 274–8.

Chapter 4 ————————————————————

Nutrition and Metabolism in the Elderly

M. R. P. HALL

NUTRITION

Introduction

The Oxford English Dictionary defines nutrition as 'the action or process of supplying or of receiving nourishment.' In discussing the subject of nutrition in the elderly we have to solve the problem of whether that nourishment is appropriate to the elderly individual. Since each individual will differ in a whole range of parameters it is only possible to give general guidelines based on studies of the dietary and energy intakes of large numbers of subjects. These dietary surveys have given us a great deal of information with regard to what and how much people eat. However, they cannot assess nutritional status: this can only be judged from clinical examination aided by laboratory findings. By then relating these findings to intake, we can judge the appropriateness of the nourishment.

Dietary surveys

The objective of a dietary survey is to find out what people eat, whether this is too much or too little, and if the balance of the constituents of the diet maintains health. A dietary survey produces information related to intake in terms of protein, fat and carbohydrate, from which the energy value of the diet can be calculated, together with the vitamin content, the amount of essential elements such as calcium and potassium, and trace elements such as zinc or copper. Clinical examination and laboratory tests will then reveal excesses or deficiencies in the diet. A diet with a higher than necessary energy intake will, for instance, lead to obesity, while a diet deficient in vitamin C will lead to scurvy – as was discoverd by Lind in the eighteenth century. In performing dietary surveys, four methods have been used.

1. Chemical analysis of the food eaten

This is without doubt the most accurate method. It is, however, time-consuming, laborious and expensive. Two identical diets have to be prepared. One is eaten, the other analysed so that the amount eaten can be estimated. Any food not eaten can also be quantified and subtracted from the total to give the amount ingested. Obviously this type of survey is more easily done in an institution such as a hospital or old people's home. It is very difficult to do in the domestic situation. This raises the question as to the value of such surveys, since they tend to be conducted only in institutional settings and old people in institutions are hardly typical of the 'normal' old person. Recently, however, studies have been successfully undertaken in the homes of fit healthy individuals (Bunker et al., 1982).

2. Dietary histories

Dietary histories of food eaten during a fixed period (usually one week) are obtained by interview. This method obviously relies on the individual's memory and depends on the skill of the interviewer. Differences will occur between interviewers, but the method may give good results if a single interviewer is used so that 'observer bias' is eliminated.

3. Recall of food eaten during the past 24 hours (24-hour recall)

This is repeated on several different occasions, but again depends on the individual's memory; and it is well recognised that short-term memory tends to decline with age and is lost early in senile dementia. Macleod (1972) however suggests that this method is simple in the elderly, and identifies more people with sub-optimal diets than the seven-day history.

4. Weighed dietary record

This is kept over a varying interval of time and often repeated more than once. Individuals participating in a survey were supplied with scales and instructed in their use. The method was used in the DHSS (Government) Surveys of 1967/8 and 1972/3 (DHSS 1972, 1979) and seems to give reasonably accurate results.

Variations and combinations of these last three methods have been widely used. They all rely on the use of food tables for estimating intake but these can only offer a representative guide with regard to the value of a particular food. They do not have the accuracy of atomic weight tables!

As can be judged from the foregoing, the study of nutrition is difficult and our knowledge is incomplete although it is increasing. The DHSS Survey (DHSS 1979) mentioned above has shown that, although intake may vary from area to area, the elderly on the whole have a smaller energy intake than the young, but the foods eaten and dietary pattern are similar. Obesity was found to be present in 24% while 7% were classified as suffering from malnutrition although the incidence was 14% in those over 80 years. The survey also showed that, while the intake of those over 80 years was less than those under 80 years, this decline was mainly due to ill health. The intake of the 'healthy' old did not vary significantly with age although men had higher intakes than women but, surprisingly, obese women were commoner in the over-80 age-group. Study of other surveys suggests that, although intake tends to fall with age, when individuals are studied over a period of years their intake remains relatively constant. Consequently it can be suggested that those with a lower intake survive longer, for the risks of obesity are well known. However, we still do not know the influence that dietary composition and intake has on longevity (Exton-Smith 1980). Some clear facts, though, have emerged from study of nutritional surveys.

Medical and social risk factors

Various dietary surveys linked to medical and social assessment have indicated clearly both positive and negative factors affecting food intake (Table 4.1). However, even though such evidence is clear, it still remains doubtful whether a factor associated with a poor intake is the cause of the poor intake or a result of it. For instance, 'being housebound' will cause a reduction in intake as the individual will not be able to get out and purchase all the food needed. On the other hand, diminished activity will reduce the need for food intake. In attempting to make judgements, one is therefore faced with a 'Catch 22' situation. Moreover, reduced intake is nearly always multifactorial and many of the factors are linked, such as depression and bereavement. It is not therefore

Table 4.1

Factors affecting food intake in the elderly

Factors likely to be associated with a good intake	Factors likely to be associated with a poor intake	
Physical activity	Partial gastrectomy Chronic bronchitis and emphysema Dementia Depression Dysphagia Poor dentition Salivation diminished	Physiological and medical causes
	Living alone Bereavement Being housebound	Social causes
	Ignorance Faddism Alcoholism	Other causes

surprising that researchers, while on the one hand admitting the importance of nutrition in maintaining health in old age, tend to view the topic with a certain amount of cynicism from the scientific viewpoint. As Caird (1980) has said: 'Of all the areas of research into human ageing that have been studied in depth, that of nutrition remains the most beset with myths and misconceptions.'

Table 4.2

Factors influencing nutritional status

Quality and quantity of food
Ingestion of food obtained – (mastication and swallowing)
Absorption and digestion – (malabsorption)
Requirement of body tissues (metabolism)

Factors influencing nutritional status

Table 4.1 sets out factors that affect food intake. Obviously food intake is closely related to nutritional status, but other factors also operate and these are summarised in Table 4.2.

The quality and quantity of food

The quality and quantity of food consumed will vary between individuals for a variety of reasons, including habits, preference, addiction (e.g. alcoholism), appetite, knowledge or ignorance, money, as well as the ability to obtain food and the skill to prepare it for consumption. Lack of interest in food and its preparation can easily alter both quantity and quality of diet and a habit can form which will lead to overt deficiency with clinical signs and symptoms. Shortage of money may also underlie a deficient intake, as will the ability to use money appropriately. Elderly widowers living alone may be particularly prone to deficiency states. Similarly the DHSS (1979) survey showed that people in receipt of Supplementary Benefit and in the lower social classes (III, IV and V) were more likely to eat food of poorer quality, even though energy intakes were similar. These diets tended to be deficient in vitamin C. Ignorance of food values probably played an important part in this deficiency, since a good-quality diet is not necessarily more expensive.

Ingestion of food

Mastication and swallowing are both important components of the ingestion process. The production of saliva diminishes with age, as the salivary glands become less efficient (see Chapter 2). As a result, mastication beomes less efficient and swallowing more difficult and food may often be chewed for long periods and then spat out. Eating consequently becomes a slow business and food put out on the plate becomes cold and unpalatable. This problem will be compounded by a poor dentition, and the intake of essential nutrients such as protein will be diminished. It has long been known that the proportion of solid foods ingested is closely associated with presence or absence of teeth. However, although inadequacy of the dentition alone as a primary factor causing poor nutrition is open to question, there is no doubt that it contributes to poor nutritional status.

Drugs may also reduce saliva. Diuretics and substances with anticholinergic effects are particularly liable to do this. Diuretics are the drugs most commonly prescribed to the elderly, being given to treat heart failure, hypertension, and oedema, while drugs with anticholinergic effects are given to treat depression (the tricyclic antidepressants), incontinence (propantheline, imipramine, flavoxate, emepronium) or gastrointestinal disorders (dicyclomine, propantheline).

Disorders of neuromuscular coordination may also make swallowing difficult (dysphagia). These may be associated with paralysis or dysfunction of the facial and masticatory muscles as well as those involved with the control of the tongue and pharynx. These muscles are often affected as a result of 'stroke'. Paralysis of the facial muscles will lead to food collecting in the cheek on the affected side. A dental prosthesis may sometimes be effective in preventing this, as it can also be when a lower motor neurone lesion of the VIIth nerve occurs. Neurological diseases may often also affect the bulbar muscles (pseudobulbar palsy) and make swallowing difficult, so that solids may be impossible to swallow and liquids make the patient choke. In these cases, semi-solids may be swallowed more easily.

Sufferers from Parkinson's Disease (paralysis agitans) often appear to suffer from excessive salivation, and 'dribbling' is obvious. This symptom is, in the main, due to the inability of these patients to swallow their saliva against gravity since their head, neck and upper trunk tend to be bent forward. Slow movements (hypokinesia) associated with rigidity and tremor compound the inability to swallow, thereby further reducing food intake. As a result, patients with Parkinson's Disease often suffer from subnutrition and have a poor nutritional status.

Many other disease processes may also interfere with ingestion of food. Rheumatoid arthritis may affect the temporomandibular joints, thus interfering with mastication. Breathlessness due to respiratory disease or associated with heart failure may make swallowing difficult. It has long been recognised that disability increases with age and it is hardly surprising therefore that food ingestion should diminish in this disabled group.

Taste and smell

It is often stated that the senses of taste and smell decline with age. However, soundly based information on this subject is lacking, and reports refer either to one sex or only a few cases. Loss of taste or abnormal (disagreeable) taste may be related to disease and improve with recovery. Abnormal taste patterns can certainly lead to a reduction in food intake but it is doubtful whether loss of taste or smell significantly reduces intake and leads to subnutrition.

Absorption and digestion

Some changes occur in gastro–intestinal function with ageing, probably because of mild generalised atrophy. Gastric hydrochloric acid secretion diminishes, and the finding of achlorhydria is common (Bird et. al. 1977). Figure 4.1 compares the normal appearance of the gastric mucosa in youth and age. Pancreatic lipase also diminishes but these changes probably have little effect on absorption, particularly in healthy individuals. However, when illness occurs or heart failure exists, digestion may well be impaired. In any case, the elderly should be advised to

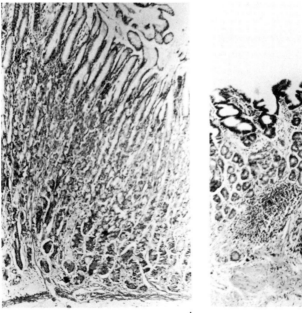

Fig 4.1a *Normal gastric mucosa in the young.*   Fig 4.1b *Normal gastric mucosa in the elderly.*

Table 4.3

Common causes of malabsorption in the elderly

Partial gastrectomy Total gastrectomy Severe atrophic gastritis 'Blind loop' syndrome	Stomach
Coeliac disease (gluten enteropathy) Jejunal diverticulosis Small bowel lymphoma	Small intestine

Drugs (anticonvulsants,
    laxatives,
    gastric irritants)	

avoid large meals and to eat smaller meals reasonably distributed during the course of the day.

Malabsorption, however, is not uncommon and may be associated with a variety of conditions in this age group (Table 4.3). The DHSS Study (1979) showed that partial gastrectomy was an important cause of subnutrition in some subjects. The other causes shown in Table 4.3 may also exist and, if present, will cause malabsorption of various nutrients. In particular, fats will be poorly absorbed in most of these conditions: vitamin D deficiency may thereby result and calcium absorption be impaired. Overgrowth of bacteria occurs in both the 'blind loop' syndrome and in jejunal diverticulosis, resulting in neutralisation of beneficial lactobacilli and deconjugation of bile salts. The same result may also occur with ageing if the gut becomes atrophied and bile secretion is grossly diminished. The condition may be cured by a broad-spectrum antibiotic such as tetracycline. Iron, folic acid and vitamin B_{12} deficiency may occur as a result of gastrectomy, chronic gastritis, or any of the small intestinal causes, as well as anticonvulsant therapy, resulting in anaemia.

It must also be remembered that disorders of the gastro-intestinal tract may give rise to nutritional or nutrient deficiency because of the loss of nutrient. Loss of iron as a result of bleeding is the commonest cause of iron deficiency anaemia in the elderly While this may occur from ulcerative lesions, neoplasms or haemorrhoids, the place of drugs – particularly gastric irritants –

must not be forgotten. Many elderly patients have their arthritis treated with aspirin or other non-steroidal anti-inflammatory drugs, and all of these may cause blood-loss from the gut. Similarly, other lesions may have other effects, e.g. potassium loss from a colonic polyp.

Finally it should be remembered that gut motility impaired by age may have effects on nutritional intake. Current fashion is to correct constipation by increasing the fibre content of the diet. While this is undoubtedly effective in increasing stool bulk, iron, calcium and magnesium ions may become attached to fibre and thus not absorbed, thereby creating deficiency. Large quantities of fibre should, therefore, not be prescribed.

Requirement of body tissues

The nutritional requirement of individual body tissues in old age is not known, but it probably declines. Certainly it seems likely that total body requirements are reduced. Both height and weight tend to diminish after the fourth decade, but there is wide variation, though after the sixth decade nearly all are affected. It is sometimes suggested that this overall reduction in body size is because those who are obese die at a younger age. However, the prevalence and degree of obesity seems to be the same at 70 years as at 50 years. Both muscle and bone mass gradually reduce with age. Maximal physical performance occurs at about 30 years, when strength and endurance are at their peak. After this a steady decline occurs, more rapidly in those who are inactive, though training can restore function and mass to the levels of active controls.

As a result of the loss of tissue, Body Cell Mass (BCM) or Lean Body Mass (LBM) is reduced and Body Fat (BF) increases. BCM declines more rapidly in men than in women. The changes in the BCM/BF ratio will alter (increase) the amount of protein required in kg/body weight. However, this is slightly offset by the reduction in extracellular fluid (ECF) which occurs. It can, however, be said that protein requirement relates directly to BCM. As a result the basal metabolic rate (BMR) will also fall. However, the fall in BMR may also be in part due to inactivity (as of course may be the fall in BCM).

It is also likely that some changes take place within tissue cells. Some enzymal patterns alter, either because protein replication is defective or because enzyme adaptability and induction is depressed or delayed. Cell sensitivity may diminish, possibly due to deficiency of target-cell receptors. This may explain reduced glucose tolerance in the elderly.

Nutritional energy intake

The nutritional surveys already referred to, as well as other cross-sectional studies relating to energy intake in various age cohorts, show that energy intake diminishes with age in both sexes. Considerable variation exists within age groups, depending on different factors such as activity, social class, habit and custom, and type of work. Table 4.4 gives examples of energy intake and it can be seen from this that intake in 75–90-year-old Edinburgh women was similar to that of women aged 25–34 in America while, in America, intake of both men and women fell steadily. The reasons why intake may decline with age have already been discussed (see Table 2.1). Nutritional deficiency is

Table 4.4

Examples of energy intake in relation to age, location and occupation

Age	Males *kcals/day	Females *kcals/day	Source
20–24	2888	1691	US National Centre for
25–34	2739	1638	Health Statistics Dietary
35–44	2554	1558	Intake Findings
45–54	2301	1533	United States 1971–74
55–64	2076	1382	
65–74	1805	1307	
62–74	2494	1771	
75–90	2176	1648	Edinburgh (1975)
22 (Students)	3060		
36 (Coal miners)	4030		
60 (Heavy work)	3430		
56 (Clerks)	2440		Scotland (1964)
21 (Shop assistants)		2200	
60 (Housewives)		1940	
70–97	2117		Cambridgeshire
71–86		1747	DHSS Survey 1979

*1 kcal≈4.2 J

common in elderly subjects admitted to hospital, and geriatricians have long recognised that many debilitated subjects re-
cover when just given good food and water. Indeed it must
be recognised that, while intake diminishes with illness, the
need for increased intake actually rises. How to increase intake
sufficiently to meet the added requirement, in the face of absence
of the desire to eat, is a major problem.

Energy and protein requirements

The requirements for protein and essential amino acids are
extremely difficult to evaluate. Those studies that have been
done have produced conflicting results (Werner 1983).
Moreover, studies are themselves difficult to evaluate since the
groups studied and the methods used are often not comparable.
It would seem likely that most healthy elderly subjects have
protein and essential amino acid requirements similar to the
young although, as suggested above, their energy needs may be
lower and they may consequently take, and perhaps need, a high
percentage of their intake in the form of protein. Certainly some
of the lower albumin levels found in old age may be directly
related to a reduced protein intake. Another possible explanation
is that this may be due to increased requirements but this is
doubtful, although it may be a result of impaired albumin
homeostasis or synthesis.

Dietary requirements, therefore, may be higher than is generally thought or recommended by national health authorities. The
recommended daily allowance (RDA) is 50–60g/day for men and
45–50g/day for women (0.7–0.8g per kg body weight). Dietary
surveys have shown that in fact elderly subjects frequently take
much more than this. Protein synthesis and breakdown (i.e.
turnover) is lower in younger people than the old and albumin
synthesis may be unaltered by changes in protein intake in the
elderly, unlike the situation in the young adult.

In disease states, however, protein requirements may be
doubled or trebled and there is no doubt that many ill old people,
unless in receipt of supplementary feeds, are considerably undernourished. This need for additional protein (and therefore essential amino acids) may occur as a result of infections, which cause
pyrexia and thereby increase metabolic rate. It may also result
from protein loss occurring from gastro-intestinal disease (e.g.
bleeding), exudate from an ulcer, pressure sore or wound, renal

lesion, surgical operation or other trauma. When the elderly do adapt successfully to protein withdrawal or loss, this is most likely to be at the expense of their own protein and consequently lean body mass. Supplementing the diet with appropriate protein and essential amino acids might well lead to better tissue repair and consequently more rapid recovery.

Little specific work has been done relating to essential amino acid needs and no clear evidence exists as to these requirements. The work that has been done suggests a higher need, but it is not certain whether this results from more rapid utilisation due to tissue repair/breakdown or whether it reflects reduced efficiency of conversion to appropriate product.

Protein balance studies suggest that a protein intake of 0.8g/kg/day is sufficient to maintain a positive nitrogen balance. Approximately 12–14% of the energy requirements should be provided as protein. Since these figures have been calculated in terms of egg protein it is probably reasonable to suggest a protein intake of 1g/kg/day. If this represents 14% of the energy requirements, total intake would be approximately 8500 joules. This represents an energy intake higher than the RDA (see above) but very similar to that found in healthy active elderly (Bunker et al. 1982). When ill, additional protein is needed. Simple disease can result in the loss of 0.3kg of body protein over several days, while a fractured femur will increase this loss to 0.7kg.

Figure 4.2 attempts to summarise in a diagrammatic form the foregoing text. In the normal individual the model will be in balance and the amino-acid pool, replenished by the intake of nutrient, will provide the materials to resynthesise protein being broken down by normal 'wear and tear,' thereby repairing body tissues. This may be interfered with by defective protein synthesis and increased breakdown. If, in addition to this, supply of nutrient is deficient and proteins are also lost, it is obvious that both amino-acid pool and body protein will diminish. Replacement, unless tackled early, will be difficult.

The assessment of nutritional state

The assessment of the general nutritional state of the elderly individual can be difficult, because different investigators will have different views of what constitutes a particular nutritional state. A single observer looking at a group of people will be able

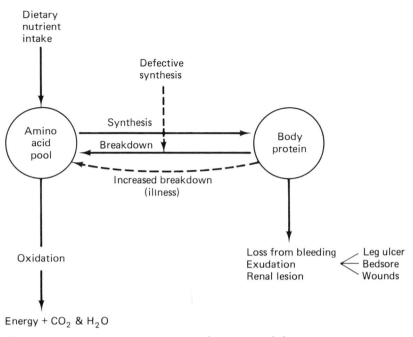

Fig 4.2   *Diagrammatic representation of protein metabolism.*

to identify those who are fat, normal, or thin according to his opinion (Table 4.5). In this study of elderly people living in the north-east of England, subjects were divided into those living alone and those living with others. In both cases there were significantly more fat women than men; the proportion of normal and thin men and women was similar, though there were slightly more thin men living alone. It might be concluded from this study that men are more likely to be undernourished than women or that old women are fatter than men. However, thinness does not necessarily mean that an individual is suffering from nutritional deficiency, although this may be an indication. Another explanation might be that obesity is a more lethal condition in men than in women. There is also some evidence that obese women have a lower energy intake than controls. Probably immobility causes a positive energy balance despite the low intake. Such people, particularly if housebound, may well suffer from nutritional deficiency in spite of appearing well nourished! Nutritional deficiency can take many forms and, as a result, many different measures can be used, from various body

Table 4.5

Nutritional state in subjects living alone and with others

		Total Number			Percentage		
		M	F	T	M	F	T
Subjects	Thin	11	46	57	23	18	19
living	Fat	0	34	34	0	13.3	11
alone	Normal	37	175	212	77	68.6	70
Subjects	Thin	52	73	125	18.7	17	17.6
living	Fat	12	77	89	4.2	18	12.5
with	Normal	214	282	496	77.1	65	69.9
others							
Total		326	687	1013	100	100	100

measurements (anthropometric) to individual nutrients (e.g. vitamins, iron).

Anthropometry

As a result of the DHSS report on Nutrition and Health in Old Age a considerable amount of information concerning body measurements has been recorded. However, it was significant that as far as obesity was concerned the observer's opinion correlated very well indeed ($P<0.001$) with Quetelet's Index, the four-site skinfold thickness, two-site and four-site percentage body fat calculations. The anthropometric parameters used in this study are shown in Table 4.6. Skinfold thickness is measured using Harpenden calipers and the mean of three measurements is usually calculated. Arm circumference is usually measured in the left upper arm at the midpoint between the acromion and the olecranon. The value of these measurements in assessing nutritional state needs, however, to be taken in context with other aspects of the individual as well as physiological, medical, environmental and genetic factors. Nutritional status will to a certain extent depend on previous development, physical activity and social status, as well as present existence, while requirements are in turn dependent on body size and composition.

While overnutrition leading to increase in body size has many dangers for the elderly, it is the diagnosis of undernutrition which taxes the clinician most. The DHSS survey mentioned above showed that 31% of the women and 17% of the men were

Table 4.6

Anthropometric indices

2-site skinfold thickness (mm) = sum of triceps and subscapular measurements

4-site skinfold thickness (mm) = sum of biceps, triceps, subscapular and suprailiac measurements

Quetelet's Index $= \dfrac{\text{Weight (kg)}}{\text{Height (m)}^2}$

Percentage body fat 2 sites

for men $= \dfrac{\left[35.685 \times \log_{10} (\text{2-site skinfold measurement (mm)})\right] - 23.715}{1.1527 - \left[0.0793 \times \log_{10} (\text{2-site skinfold measurement (mm)})\right]}$

for women $= \dfrac{\left[33.39 \times \log_{10} (\text{2-site skinfold measurement (mm)})\right] - 15.615}{1.1347 - \left[0.0742 \times \log_{10} (\text{2-site skinfold measurement (mm)})\right]}$

Percentage body fat 4 sites

for men $= \dfrac{\left[35.055 \times \log_{10} (\text{4-site skinfold measurement (mm)})\right] - 32.175}{1.1715 - \left[0.0779 \times \log_{10} (\text{4-site skinfold measurement (mm)})\right]}$

for women $= \dfrac{\left[29.025 \times \log_{10} (\text{4-site skinfold measurement (mm)})\right] - 15.255}{1.1339 - \left[0.0645 \times \log_{10} (\text{4-site skinfold measurement (mm)})\right]}$

Arm muscle area (cm²) $= \dfrac{\left[\text{Area circumference (mm)} - \pi \times \text{Triceps (mm)}\right]^2}{400\,\pi}$

Lean arm radius (mm) $= \dfrac{\left[\text{Arm circumference (mm)}\right] - \left[\text{Triceps (mm)} \times 0.6\right]}{2\,\pi}$

obese, while only 7% of the sample had evidence of subnutrition. From this it would appear that we should, perhaps, be more concerned with overnutrition; that we are not is probably because we recognise subnutrition as a condition linked to disease, both caused by it and causing it. Emphasis has been placed particularly on the diagnosis of subnutrition in the management of the surgical patient, and the assessment of the nutritional state with regard to surgical management has been recognised as

Table 4.7

Score card for protein malnutrition

Weight loss	Greater than 10% of ideal weight
Mid-triceps skinfold thickness	Less than 10mm (men); 13mm (women)
Mid-triceps arm muscle circumference	Less than 23cm (men); 22cm (women)
Lymphocyte count	Less than 1 500/microlitre
Serum albumin	Less than 35g/l
Serum transferrin	Less than 2g/l
Impairment of cellular immunity	Impaired response to skin test(s) for delayed hypersensitivity (e.g. to tuberculin)

important. A score card for protein malnutrition has been devised (Table 4.7), and it has been suggested that patients who score badly should be specially prepared for and treated during surgery with nutritional supplements which will enable them to withstand trauma and heal more quickly. This lead given by surgical colleagues has not always been followed by geriatricians or physicians and the prescription of nutritional supplements and special diets is often ignored unless specific disease such as diabetes mellitus is diagnosed. Dietary prescription – apart from the routine prescription of vitamins – seems to be the responsibility of the ward sister and her nursing staff rather than the dietitian or the medical staff. Yet studies have shown that mental and physical disability are related to subnutrition in elderly patients (MacLennan et al. 1975).

Diagnosis of subnutrition

Subnutrition may be defined as a disturbance of form due to lack of energy intake or of one or more nutrients (DHSS, 1979). The clinical diagnosis is, however, difficult, for there is a long latent period before the appearance of overt clinical signs resulting from a low nutrient level. Biochemical and haematological investigations may help in making the diagnosis but it is debatable whether the abnormality revealed is the result of nutrient deficiency or of an ageing change.

Table 4.7 shows some of the measurements that may be made in order to decide if protein malnutrition exists. However, skin changes occur naturally as a result of ageing changes and the parameter given here for mid-triceps skin-fold thickness is

Table 4.8

Clinical signs which may be found as a result of deficiency of nutrient

Nutrient	Clinical signs of deficiency
Vitamin A	Night blindness, neutropenia
Vitamin B complex Vitamin B1 (thiamine) Vitamin B2 (riboflavine) Vitamin B6 (pyridoxine) Nicotinic acid (niacin) Pantothenic acid	Peripheral neuropathy, Wernicke's encephalopathy, Korsakoff's psychosis, cardiac failure Angular stomatitis, cheilosis, nasolabial seborrhoea, glossitis Irritability, memory loss, headache (early) dermatitis, diarrhoea, dementia (pellagra) (late)
Vitamin B12	Megaloblastic anaemia, subacute combined degeneration of the spinal cord
Folic acid	Megaloblastic anaemia
Vitamin C	Scurvy, anaemia, weakness, delay in wound healing
Vitamin D	Osteomalacia, proximal muscle weakness, 'waddling gait'
Vitamin K	Subcutaneous haemorrhage
Iron	Atrophic glossitis, angular stomatitis, atrophic buccal mucosa, koilonychia, anaemia, reduced resistance to infection
Potassium	Muscle weakness, apathy, confusion, cardiac arrhythmia
Magnesium	Confusion, tremor, ataxia, irritability
Sodium	Weakness, postural hypotension, oedema
Calcium	Tetany
Trace elements (zinc, copper chromium, cadmium)	Delayed wound healing (zinc), anaemia (copper)

almost certainly unreliable. Moreover, it may be necessary to adjust this figure by age so that there is a different norm for the 65–74 year age group and for the over-75s. Similarly, there is a considerable loss of muscle bulk with ageing. Hence mid-triceps arm circumference may be unreliable as a measure. Arm muscle area (cm²) and lean arm radius (mm) may be better measurements. However, it should be remembered that bone is also lost. Quetelet's Index remains a useful guide but height may be difficult to measure in the elderly. Span (or half span) may be easier to measure, and correlates well with height.

Impaired cellular immunity may also occur as an ageing change. Lymphocyte counts are often low in old age so that counts below 1500/microlitre in sick old people are not uncommon, and may not indicate subnutrition. This leaves two biochemical tests. Serum transferrin levels have a wide range in the elderly and therefore may not be a reliable guide to subnutrition. More work needs to be done in this field.

Low plasma albumin is a frequent finding in nutritional surveys. However, as has already been mentioned, albumin synthesis is lower in the elderly, and the elderly may not be able to raise albumin levels if the rate of synthesis is set too low. Nevertheless this may be the most useful of the available biochemical parameters.

All these factors need to be taken into consideration in making a diagnosis of subnutrition, as indeed do the clinical and dietary history and the clinical examination. To these observations may be added measurement of specific nutrients such as the vitamins and trace elements.

Physical signs in subnutrition

Subnutrition may give rise to a variety of clinical signs. These are summarised in Table 4.8. Some of these signs relate to the mouth, while other deficiencies may interfere with wound healing. From the dental viewpoint these facts are of obvious importance.

The commonest and most important deficiencies are those relating to B complex deficiency (including vitamin B_{12} and folic acid) vitamin C, vitamin D, iron and the cations. The part that these play in causing disease in the elderly is, however, comparatively rare. In the DHSS (1979) Survey only two subjects were found to have scurvy and, although 57 were diagnosed as having either cheilosis or angular stomatitis, only four of these were found to have riboflavine deficiency. However, the subjects surveyed in this study were 'normal' elderly people and it is perhaps not surprising that deficiency was seldom detected. When it was found it was clearly associated with disease and disability. Consequently it is in this group that the physical signs of deficiency should be sought.

Vitamin B complex deficiency (including folic acid and vitamin B12)

There is doubt as to the extent to which B complex deficiency can be blamed for the lesions seen on the lips, tongue and buccal mucosa. Trials of replacement therapy have given variable results; some have shown improvement with supplementation while others have shown no improvement, leading to suggestions that the changes seen may be ascribed to fungal infections.

Thiamine status may be assessed by transketolase assay, and riboflavin and pyridoxine status can also be assessed biochemically. However, the value below which deficiency is found will be critical in determining the proportion found to be deficient. For instance Thurnham (1972) in a study of a random sample of elderly people in London found a percentage stimulation of greater than 30% of erythrocyte glutathione reductase activity by flavium adenine dinucleotide, in about 20% of the population. This indicates that marginal riboflavin deficiency may be present in one-fifth of the 'normal' elderly population.

Gross B complex deficiency is rare and usually only seen in elderly alcoholics, who may be commoner than is generally realised. The mental symptoms of Korsakoff's psychosis will respond to large doses of B complex given intravenously. The acute confusional state in the acutely ill may also be linked to a relative thiamine deficiency and it is well recognised that intravenous high-potency vitamin injection may speed recovery.

Vitamin B12 deficiency

Since vitamin B12 occurs in most animal tissues, its occurrence as a pure dietary deficiency is rare except in very strict vegetarians. It is absorbed from the ileum after binding with a mucoprotein, intrinsic factor (IF), secreted by gastric parietal cells. The commonest cause of deficiency is pernicious anaemia (PA). Other causes are also linked to malabsorption and these are shown in Table 4.9.

Table 4.9

Causes of malabsorption of vitamin B12

Gastric Lesions
   Pernicious anaemia
   Atrophic gastritis
   Total gastrectomy

Intestinal Lesions
   Gluten enteropathy
   Tropical sprue
   Ileal resection or disease (Crohn's disease)
   Abnormal small gut bacterial flora (jejunal diverticulosis, blind loop
      syndrome, fistula)
   Pancreatic disease
   Drug-induced malabsorption (phenytoin)
   Fish tapeworm

Folic acid deficiency

Megaloblastic anaemia associated with folate deficiency is not uncommon and is associated with malabsorption, liver disease (particularly associated with alcoholism), and a low intake; folates occur in fresh green vegetables, nuts, yeast and liver. The incidence in the elderly has been overemphasised, partly because of inappropriate sampling of elderly subjects, partly because too high a 'cut-off' point has been taken to indicate normality, and partly because serum levels have been taken as the indicator. Serum folate levels are difficult to evaluate because dietary folate deficiency present for only a short time can lower serum levels to an apparently critical level without depleting tissue stores. Such deficiency may be transient and red blood cell folate levels are a much better indicator of true tissue folate deficiency. Even so, levels below 150 μg/l (normal range 150–600 μg/l) packed red cells are not uncommon, and surveys indicate a prevalence of between 8–16% (DHSS (1972)).

Table 4.10

Vitamin C intake expressed as a percentage of RDA

Men		Women	
65–74 years	75 years +	65–74 years	75 years +
143	127	133	113

Vitamin C deficiency

The classical condition of scurvy is still seen but is rare. It is commoner in old men but may also occur in hospitalised patients who are not supplemented. The RDA for vitamin C is 30mg/day. The DHSS survey (1979) showed that the majority had a higher intake though this tended to drop with age (Table 4.10). However some special sub-groups existed whose intake was lower; these were subjects with a low mental test score, in the lower social classes (IV and V), or in receipt of supplementary benefit.

It is generally agreed that a daily intake of 10mg of ascorbic acid will prevent scurvy though, in order to maintain a leucocyte ascorbic acid (LAA) level of $15\mu g/10^8$ cells, the daily intake may need to be 11.3mg for men and 16.3mg for women.

Vitamin C status can be assessed by measuring ascorbic acid levels in plasma, leucocytes or whole blood. Many studies have shown that low levels are found in different samples of the elderly. Most of these measure LAA levels and a content of $15\mu g/10^8$ white cells was taken as the lower limit of normal. However there seems to be little relation between LAA levels and vitamin C intake, though LAA levels will rise if supplements of vitamin C are given. There is also a seasonal variation, with levels being higher in the second half of the year.

The significance of a low LAA level is doubtful, unless it is very low and overt scurvy is present. It is also possible that low levels of LAA are an indicator of illness rather than ascorbic acid deficiency. It has been shown that patients in hospital with levels less than $12\mu g/10^8$ cells had a significantly higher mortality than patients with a level of over $25\mu g/10^8$ cells ($P<0.01$). This finding was not related to the LAA level but to the severity of the illness, and administration of vitamin C did not influence mortality nor increase LAA levels (Wilson et al. 1973). Moreover, LAA levels show an inverse relationship with the polymorphonuclear leucocyte count, so that low levels are associated with leucocytosis.

The whole topic requires further study and it may be that ascorbic acid plasma levels, alone or linked with saturation tests, will prove better for evaluating the vitamin C status of the elderly (Thomas et al. 1984).

Certainly in the DHSS (1979) study the plasma ascorbic acid (PAA) seemed a more valuable measure than the LAA in assessing vitamin C status. Levels of PAA of less than 0.2mg/100ml were significant in subjects with poor dentition ($P<0.05$), who were wasted ($P<0.05$), who smoked ($P<0.01$) and who were in receipt of supplementary benefit ($P<0.05$).

Vitamin D deficiency

Vitamin D deficiency causes a generalised decalcification of bone matrix known as osteomalacia. It is multifactorial in origin (Table 4.11). Patients initially complain of vague pains which are often dismissed as 'rheumatism'. These persist, however, and as they become more localised bones may become tender. Muscular weakness may be marked so that difficulty is experienced when climbing stairs or standing from the sitting position. It is most marked in the proximal muscles of the shoulders and pelvis. The radiological appearance of the spine shows kyphosis with an increased concavity of the intervertebral disc spaces ('cod-fish vertebrae'). Looser's zones (pseudofractures), consisting of an area of translucency bordered by a band of dense callus, may be seen in various sites such as upper ends of femora, the pubic rami, the ribs and the scapular border.

Patients with osteomalacia will also show changes in some biochemical parameters. Alkaline phosphatase is raised, and

Table 4.11

Possible causes of osteomalacia in old age

Low dietary intake of vitamin D
Lack of exposure to sunlight
Malabsorption syndromes
Increased physiological requirement of vitamin D
Impaired conversion of vitamin D to 25-OH D3 in liver
Impaired conversion of 25-OH D3 to 1,25 dihydroxycholecalciferol in kidney

electrophoresis will distinguish this rise as coming from bone; serum calcium will be low, as will phosphorus. The 25-hydroxycholecalciferol (25-OH D3) level will also be low, and parathyroid hormone levels will be higher than normal making the diagnosis of primary hyperparathyroidism difficult. Levels of 25-OH D3 tend to be lower in the sick or institutionalised elderly, and the distribution of levels in the fit elderly is similar to that found in the young (Fig. 4.3). This is presumably because the ill elderly not only eat a poorer diet but also tend to be housebound and therefore do not go out in the sun.

Vitamin K deficiency

Vitamin K is primarily concerned with the synthesis of four coagulation factors – prothrombin and Factors VII, IX and X. It occurs as either phylloquinone (vitamin K1) or menoquinones (vitamin K2), and its absorption from the small intestine is dependent on bile salts. Consequently, deficiency occurs in obstructive jaundice. It is very rare as a nutritional deficiency.

Iron deficiency

In health, iron requirement is low, being that amount needed to replace mean daily loss – 0.6mg daily. The RDA however is much higher than this, being 10mg daily to allow a wide margin of safety (DHSS 1969). Iron deficiency in the elderly is common, but it may not always give rise to anaemia. The symptoms and signs of iron deficiency are listed in Table 4.8. To these may be added fatigue, lassitude and pallor. The onset may be insidious and is sometimes attributed to 'getting old' so that the deficiency is not recognised until some other complication such as heart failure or mental confusion ensues.

The commonest cause of iron deficiency is blood loss, though dietary deficiency can occur and absorption of iron may also be impaired. In some conditions, iron requirements may be increased so that a relative deficiency occurs in, e.g. chronic anoxia, polycythaemia, or chronic haemolysis. The commonest site of blood loss is the gastrointestinal tract. Haemorrhoids are probably the commonest cause, though gastric bleeding associated with hiatus hernia or erosions due to aspirin and other non-steroidal anti-inflammatory drugs (NSAIDs) must now be nearly as common. Peptic ulceration, carcinoma of stomach or

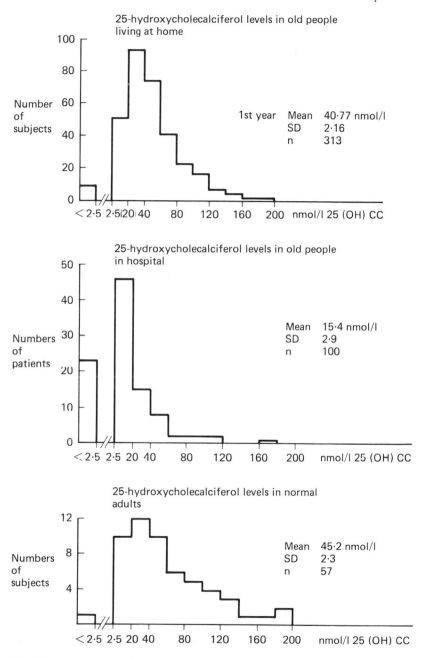

Fig 4.3   *Comparison of vitamin D levels in young, fit elderly, and old people in hospital.*

large bowel, and diverticular disease are also common causes. Other causes such as oesophageal varices, coloproctitis and rectal carcinoma are less common causes of iron deficiency in old age.

Diagnosis of iron deficiency is not usually difficult since the blood picture is usually that of a hypochromic, microcytic anaemia. The serum iron is low ($<9\mu$mol/l) and the total iron-binding capacity (TIBC) is high ($>71\mu$mol/l). However, the TIBC tends to fall in old age and is often lowered together with the serum iron in the 'anaemia of chronic disorders' which is so common in old age. Estimation of serum iron and TIBC may therefore be of doubtful value and a therapeutic trial of oral iron may be a better way of clinching the diagnosis, combined with investigation of the faeces for occult blood.

Treatment should be aimed at eliminating the cause, e.g. by stopping aspirin or other NSAIDs, treating peptic ulcer or removing a carcinoma, and giving iron by mouth. This may be combined with ascorbic acid since this improves iron absorption. Most cases respond but those that do not will require further investigation. Bone marrow examination will confirm the presence of stores of iron, i.e. whether there is a utilisation block; an absorption test will show if iron is absorbed, and may also help to distinguish malabsorption from failure of the patient to comply with treatment. If oral iron is unsuccessful then it may be necessary to resort to intramuscular injections or even blood transfusion.

Potassium deficiency

Many elderly people have a diet that is deficient in potassium. An average normal diet contains 50–150mmol/day. Judge (1980) suggests that 60mmol/day is probably generous and yet many elderly do not achieve this; a random sample of population has shown that 9% of men and 14% women take less than 40mmol daily. In addition to this low intake, excess loss of potassium is common. This is mainly due to reduced renal tubular reabsorption, often resulting from treatment with diuretics, which are amongst the most commonly used drugs. Depletion may also occur, however, in sodium retention syndromes such as hyperaldosteronism, Cushing's syndrome, overdosage with corticosteroids or carbenoxolone, acidosis, hyperchloraemia and potassium-losing nephropathies. Potassium may also be lost as a result of vomiting and diarrhoea, from mucous loss in the spurious diarrhoea of faecal impaction, as a consequence of tumours of the rectum and large bowel, and alimentary fistulae.

Potassium deficiency causes muscle weakness, apathy, confusion, abdominal distension, paralytic ileus, constipation, cardiac arrhythmias, and reduced cardiac output and failure with oedema. This may lead to more diuretic being given and cardiac failure being treated with digitalis, with interaction and unwanted drug effect. Moreover acute depletion may occur due to sudden migration of ion during treatment of severe anaemia, particularly pernicious anaemia, or of diabetic coma.

Awareness of the common prevalence of potassium deficiency and its seriousness is most important. Treatment with oral potassium supplements is essential. It is important to remember that proprietary preparations only contain small amounts and it is often necessary to give supplements of the order of 80–100 moles daily; occasionally, intravenous supplementation is necessary, but the rate should not exceed 20mmol per hour.

It is worth remembering that potassium retention gives rise to almost the same symptomatology. Awareness of the risk of deficiency leads to the use of potassium-sparing diuretics. If these are used in the presence of renal failure or given in conjunction with potassium supplements then retention of potassium and cardiac arrest may occur.

Calcium deficiency

Skeletal calcium diminishes steadily with age, and the rate increases in some women after the menopause. As a result the incidence of fractures increases with age and this is related in particular to fractures of the lower forearm (Colles' fracture), compression fractures of vertebrae, and fractures of the upper end of the femur. There is no doubt that all these fractures are associated with an increasing incidence of osteoporosis, and it would appear that trabecular bone is affected at an earlier age than cortical bone so that fractures of the upper end of the femur occur in an older age group. Calcium and hormonal deficiency in women may contribute towards the development of osteoporosis.

The role of dietary calcium deficiency, however, is probably slight. The DHSS (1979) Survey showed that the calcium intake in all subjects was more than one-and-a-half times the calcium RDA. However, vitamin D intake in the women was lower than the RDA. Since 1,25 dihydroxycholecalciferol (1,25-(OH)$_2$D3) is necessary for calcium absorption, and since conversion of 25-OH D3 to 1,25-(OH)$_2$D3 may be impaired, absorption of calcium may also be diminished. As a result, an element of osteomalacia may coexist with the osteoporosis, and histological evidence of osteomalacia may be found in 25% of cases with femoral neck fracture. This probably explains some of the conflicting evidence on calcium supplementation and its effect on osteoporosis and bone mass. Despite claims that 800mg daily of elemental calcium delays bone loss, a calcium intake of 1000–2000mg daily was found to be ineffective in preventing bone loss over a two-year period in the early menopause (Nilas et al. 1984). In a review of the literature, Werner (1983) states that reports of restitution of normal bone with calcium therapy have not been convincing. One such report claims the reversal of localised osteoporosis in periodontal disease with extra calcium (Lutwak et al. 1971).

Treatment of osteoporosis therefore remains difficult. Probably the most rational regime is a combination of a low-dose oestrogen such as mestranol with 1α-OH D3 in a dose of 1μg daily.

As has already been mentioned, calcium and vitamin D are intricately related, and linked to parathyroid hormone excretion. Absence of parathyroid hormone causes catastrophic calcium deficiency, and the low calcium levels give rise to tetany. This can be diagnosed clinically by the occurrence of carpopedal spasm. The parathyroid glands may be damaged after thyroidectomy but otherwise would appear to function normally. Also associated with hypoparathyroidism is an increased incidence of cataract.

Magnesium deficiency

Like potassium, magnesium deficiency is common in old age, with many elderly people taking diets deficient in this element. Absorption is similar to that of calcium although vitamin D is not necessary. High fibre diets may prevent absorption and diuretics may increase urinary loss. Symptoms include weakness, ataxia, tremor and confusion, and can be relieved by oral supplements which may, of course, cause purgation and further loss!

Sodium deficiency

Sodium deficiency is not uncommon in debilitated sick elderly people. It may often result from dietary deficiency linked with diuretic therapy. One of the most worrying symptoms is postural (orthostatic) hypotension, which gives rise to loss of confidence, dizziness and falls. As a result the patient remains bedfast which in itself causes further sodium depletion. Increased intake of salt may correct the condition but salt retention may have to be induced by giving a fluorinated steroid (fludrocortisone) in a dose of 0.1mg daily.

Trace elements

Comparatively little is as yet known about the role of trace elements in the elderly. It can be hypothesised that accumulation of some substances such as lead and cadmium and deficiency of others such as zinc, chromium and copper may be harmful. Recently Bunker et al. (1984a) have studied the intake and excretion of lead and cadmium in healthy elderly people living in their own homes. They found these subjects to be in negative balance and not at risk of accumulating these toxic metals. In a similar study the same group (Bunker et al. 1984b) have investigated the uptake and excretion of chromium. It has been suggested that impaired glucose tolerance and ischaemic heart disease may be secondary to chromium deficiency, and both conditions are common in the elderly. However, although the subjects studied by Bunker and her colleagues had a chromium intake below the lower limit of RDA proposed by the American Food and Nutrition Board, they were in dietary equilibrium or slight positive balance. It would seem therefore that a low intake in these subjects may be acceptable but it may not be sufficient to meet situations when requirements are raised or losses increased.

Zinc deficient diets in the institutionalised elderly and in the elderly at home are common. This may account for the decreased plasma zinc levels found in this age group even in a relatively 'normal' population. It is not certain what effect this has but zinc supplementation to promote wound healing can certainly be justified on theoretical grounds. (Bunker et al. 1982).

METABOLISM

Many of the metabolic problems that are met in the elderly have already been discussed when considering nutrition. The links between anaemia and iron and vitamins, and bone disorders and vitamin D and calcium are examples, while the influence of some of the endocrine glands and of renal function have been hinted at. This part of the chapter will therefore consider in a little more detail the effect of age on the endocrine system; finally a discussion on the metabolism of drugs will illustrate further the effect of age on absorption, hepatic metabolism and excretion.

Endocrine system

The ability to respond or adjust to stress declines with age. Since the endocrine system can be shown to be associated with the adjustment of the body to stress and shock as well as 'flight and fight', many authors have proposed that changes will occur in the function and structure of the component parts of the system. Indeed it has been suggested that ageing is regulated by the hypothalamic–hypophysoperipheral endocrine system and the presence of an 'ageing clock' mechanism situated in the hypothalamus has been postulated. The evidence for this, however, is conflicting. Patients with Simmonds' disease (due to pituitary deficiency) appear prematurely old, yet such deficiency has never been shown to occur in the premature ageing conditions such as progeria and Werner's syndrome. Moreover, patients with Cushing's syndrome (hypercorticoadrenalism) also show features of premature ageing. Yet in animals prednisolone may prolong life-span and hypophysectomy may retard bone ageing.

The foregoing suggests that there is no simple answer. Indeed when one considers the loose structure of the endocrine system and the many factors, including diseases, which may affect it (Fig. 4.4) this is not surprising. Man is hardly the easiest of experimental animals to study.

Hypophysoadrenal system

There would seem to be little difference between the histological appearance of either hypophysis or adrenal with age though it is likely, in common with other organs, that their cell membranes

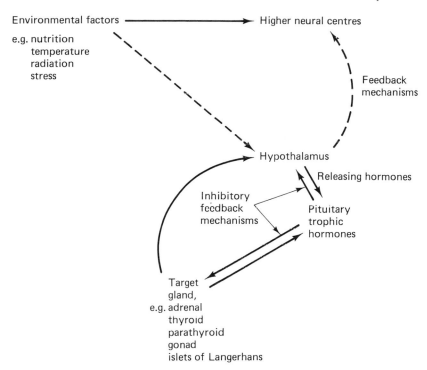

Fig 4.4   *The relationship between various components of the neuro-endocrine system.*

may be less permeable. There may also be an increase in fibrous tissue, some loss of basophilic cells, and a tendency for adenomas to be more common in both pituitary and adrenal.

Both glands, however, respond well to tests designed to provoke maximal hormonal secretion. It might be expected that growth hormone (GH) secretion is diminished with ageing but the subjects – aged 82–95 years – studied by Cartlidge et al. (1970) showed a normal response to insulin-induced hypoglycaemia. All the evidence available therefore seems to indicate that the hypothalamic–hypophysoadrenal system functions well in fit elderly people. Blichert-Toft (1975) has reviewed the literature and studied the response to surgical stress in a group of patients aged 65–86 years. He found that adrenocorticotrophic hormone (ACTH) release was normal, but that GH response was more variable in the old when compared with the young, and that it would appear to be dissociated from ACTH response. He felt that routine postoperative tests of hypothalamic–hypophysoadrenal function were unnecessary but that they might be of value in chronically ill patients or those already on steroid therapy. Additional groups of patients who may have diminished function are those with severe subnutrition and depression. However, as already noted, these groups may be intermingled with the chronically ill.

Finally, cortisone and its derivatives are used therapeutically in elderly patients in a variety of conditions. Decreased cortisone utilisation occurs in the old, so that the half-life is prolonged. Consequently blood levels may be high and iatrogenic hypercorticoadrenalism may result.

The posterior pituitary or neurohypophysis, like the anterior gland and the adrenal cortex and medulla, remains relatively unaffected by the ageing process. Recently, however, there has been some evidence to suggest that vasopressin levels increase with age. It is possible that this may relate to the increase in blood pressure seen with age.

The signs and symptoms of hypo- or hyperfunction of the hypophysoadrenal axis are well described in the standard text books. These do not differ significantly in the elderly. It is worth remembering that, as a result of true ageing, many elderly may display symptoms and show features which could be attributed to altered function. These features include increased pigmentation, pallor, loss of body iron, hypotension, lethargy and mental confusion – all of which may be associated with hypofunction; obesity, plethora, hypertension and osteoporosis may indicate hyperfunction. It is important therefore to maintain a 'high index of suspicion' if the patient's response to standard treatments is abnormal.

The thyroid gland and the hypophysothyroid axis

Hypo- and hyperfunction of the thyroid gland is common in the elderly population, with hypofunction being the commoner.

Hypothyroidism (myxoedema) can be found in between 2–3% of admissions of elderly people to hospital (Jeffreys, 1972). In some of these, the diagnosis would not have been suspected on clinical grounds alone. Symptoms of the condition include obesity, mental and physical slowing, deafness or cold intolerance, and loss of hair, all of which could be attributed to growing old as, indeed, they often (mistakenly) are. The gruff voice may not always be present, and slow relaxation of the ankle jerk or other reflexes may be missed or not tested for. Similarly, constipation is common in the immobile elderly, while limb pains may be mistaken for 'rheumatism', 'arthritis', or bone pain. A recent study of 347 elderly people living in their own homes revealed four cases of hypothyroidism being treated and another nine cases that had not been diagnosed, giving a total prevalence of 3.7% (Southampton Ageing Project).

Such a high pick-up of cases means that all health professionals need to be on the lookout for this condition and should not accept apparent ageing signs without first excluding hypothyroidism. This may be done by estimating the 'free T4' in blood. If this value is low – below 9pmol/l – then the thyroid-stimulating hormone (TSH) levels should be measured. TSH is secreted by the anterior hypophysis, with the normal range being from 0.8–3.5μm/l.

However, it is generally accepted that levels vary between laboratories and that TSH levels tend to rise with age. Levels up to 5μm/l may therefore be acceptable as 'normal' for the elderly, and levels as high as 6μm/l may not always be abnormal. If the TSH is raised in conjunction with a low 'free T4', the diagnosis of primary thyroid failure can be made. If, however, the TSH level is low and hypothyroidism is still suspected, then thyrotrophin-releasing hormone (TRH) should be given as a single intravenous injection of 400μg or as an oral dose of 20–40mg. This will be followed by a rise in TSH, tri-iodothyronine (T3) and thyroxine (T4). However this will not happen if there is hypophyseal failure. This test is known as the TRH-stimulation test and may also help to distinguish those borderline cases with a low T4 and a high normal TSH since a sustained rise in TSH, T3, and T4 will occur.

Treatment of hypothyroidism is easy since it consists of replacing the deficient hormone. Since thyroxine (T4) is converted into tri-iodothyronine (T3) in the body, it would seem rational to use T3. However, thyroxine is cheap and gives a more even level of active hormone, so that it is rarely necessary to use T3. It is wise to give thyroxine in a small dose initially, 25μg at night, doubling this after two weeks and doubling it again after a further two weeks. A dose of more than 100μg rarely needs to be used, though occasionally the dose may need increasing to 150μg.

The high prevalence of hypothyroidism is probably due to alteration of immune response in old age. Antithyroid antibody titres of over 1:25 are common in the elderly, particularly in elderly women, and may be present in as many as one in three of those aged over 85 years. This finding is not as common in men and may account for the preponderance of women with this condition.

Hyperthyroidism (thyrotoxicosis) is not as common as hypothyroidism. Jeffreys (1972) found a prevalence of 2.3% in 300 consecutive admissions to the Geriatric Unit at Northwick Park. This is much higher than has been previously reported, and may be due to the fact that thyroid function tests such as the T4 are raised in illness and may also be altered by some drugs. Nevertheless, hyperthyroidism may often be missed since its presentation may be atypical in the elderly. Rather than showing the typical signs of hyperactivity, irritability, restlessness, sweating, tachycardia, eye signs, and weight-loss in the presence of a good appetite, many elderly exhibit malaise, no eye signs, and apathy. Atrial fibrillation is common, some sufferers have heart failure, and mental confusion may occur. The condition is diagnosed by finding a high 'free T4' in the blood.

Surgical treatment is rarely necessary and patients are usually treated with radioactive iodine (^{131}I). Some patients may need treating medically with carbimazole initially.

Parathyroids

Parathyroid function is slightly depressed in normal elderly people, who have lower levels of parathyroid hormone. However, the sick elderly may often have higher than normal levels, sometimes so high that the diagnosis of primary hyperparathyroidism may prove difficult. These patients may have high serum calcium levels, and the condition may be associated with low vitamin D levels and renal disease or failure.

Gonads

Ovarian function ceases at the menopause so that female hormone levels begin to decline and the oestrogen:testosterone ratio begins to alter. This may lead to the loss of some of the secondary sexual characteristics of the female; breasts may atrophy and facial hair growth may increase. Similarly in the male, testosterone levels slowly decrease so that the testosterone:oestrogen ratio alters in the opposite direction to the female, leading to a tendency to feminisation. The effects that these hormonal changes have on metabolic functions is not clear.

Carbohydrate intolerance — diabetes mellitus

The inability to handle a glucose load increases with age so that, over the age of 70, 20% of men and 30% of women have glucose tolerance test (GTT) patterns which are compatible with a diagnosis of diabetes. The prevalence is so high as to cast doubt on the value of the GTT in the elderly. There is however no evidence to show degeneration of the islets of Langerhans in old age, and a prompt and normal insulin response to an oral glucose load occurs even in very elderly subjects (Smith and Hall 1973). It may be that receptor cells are less sensitive to the insulin produced, or that the insulin itself is less active. As a result many elderly people can be classified as suffering from maturity-onset diabetes and are therefore prone to the complications which are associated with this condition.

These complications involve the cardiovascular system, the kidney, the nervous system and the eye. Vascular complications include a retinopathy characterised by microaneurysms, blot haemorrhages, and exudates which may develop into a serious proliferative retinopathy. Coronary artery disease is also common, as is peripheral vascular disease which particularly affects the feet. Renal changes are associated with a diffuse glomerulosclerosis that causes the blood urea to rise and may, rarely, develop into a full-blown nephrotic syndrome. The changes in the nervous system result in a peripheral neuropathy which is patchy and particularly affects the sensory nerves, with patients complaining of dysaesthesia and stabbing or aching pains in the legs. In addition to this neuropathy, many elderly diabetics also suffer from autonomic dysfunction that gives rise to postural hypotension, bladder atony and bowel dysfunction, including diarrhoea and constipation. Other eye changes include an increased incidence of cataract.

The onset of diabetes in the elderly is often insidious and may be picked up as an incidental finding when the patient falls ill frequently with an infection which is often respiratory. Weight-loss may be gradual and precede diagnosis by five to ten years. Thirst may not be marked. Pruritus is common, particularly of the vulva in women, as is a flexural dermatitis that is nearly always associated with *Candida albicans* infection. Urinary tract infections are also common, and may lead to incontinence. These symptoms respond rapidly when the diabetes is brought under control.

Many elderly diabetics can be adequately treated by dietary measures controlling intake of both carbohydrate and calories. Those who cannot be so treated may be given sulphonylureas such as tolbutamide, glibenclamide or chlorpropamide, by mouth. Tolbutamide has the shortest half-life and is less likely to accumulate than chlorpropamide; hence it is probably safer to use, though it may need to be taken three times a day. Those who cannot be controlled with oral hypoglycaemics will need to be given insulin.

As has been stated earlier, many elderly people are prescribed thiazide diuretics. These are thought to inhibit insulin release and may actually increase carbohydrate intolerance so that diabetes is diagnosed. This will regress if the drug is withdrawn or will usually respond to dietary control if the diuretic has to be continued.

Drug metabolism

The incidence of sickness increases steadily with age and consequently the elderly will need medication. It is therefore important to know how drugs act in the elderly individual. Consequently much work has been done in recent years on pharmacokinetics in older people. Surveys suggest that more than 80% of elderly subjects are taking at least one medicine (see also Chapter 3), and that the prevalence of adverse reactions increases not only with age but with the number of drugs being taken.

The many physiological and biochemical changes associated with ageing alter body composition, and the efficiency of individual organs diminishes. Lean body mass is reduced and fat mass increased. Organ blood-flow is diminished. In the kidney, this will reduce glomerular filtration rate and alter body salt and water content. In the liver, metabolism may be diminished so that first-pass effect is lost. Changes in cell membrane will alter receptor functions, and numbers of receptors may be lost. Nutritional deficiency may lower plasma proteins and albumin levels, thus affecting protein binding of drugs. Many drugs are formulated as bases and we have seen that some elderly people eat a protein-deficient diet, so that they tend to excrete acid and conserve base. As a result, alkaline drugs will also be conserved and persist for a long time in the circulation. All these points must be taken into account when considering drug metabolism.

Once a drug has been prescribed it has to be taken, absorbed, metabolised in the liver, transported to the end organ, utilised and excreted. The steps in this sequence relate to compliance, absorption, hepatic metabolism, plasma transportation, tissue distribution and organ sensitivity and excretion. Each step may be altered by ageing.

a. Compliance

It is often said that the more drugs an old person has to take, the worse compliance is likely to be. A recent study (Abrams and Andrews, 1984) showed in fact that the poor compliers were those on one or two drugs, whereas those on many complied well. However, this study also showed that the elderly themselves tended actively to alter their prescribed drug regimes.

b. Absorption

This is little affected by ageing itself. However, absorption may be influenced by the action of other drugs. Laxatives, for example, may speed gastrointestinal transit so that absorption of the drug is reduced or, alternatively, other drugs (e.g. anticholinergics) may slow transit time so that absorption is increased. Drugs may also interact to form less absorbable complexes. Tetracycline and iron form a less soluble chelate.

c. Hepatic metabolism

While it has been shown in animals that enzyme induction is delayed by ageing, there is not much evidence to show that this happens in man. However, hepatic metabolism is undoubtedly less efficient for some drugs, so that higher blood levels of drug are attained. This is probably due to reduction in hepatic blood flow.

d. Plasma transport

Binding sites on plasma protein molecules, particularly albumin, are reduced with age. Consequently more free drug will be available in the case of those drugs which are highly protein-bound, e.g. warfarin, sulphonylureas. This effect, however, is likely to be transitory and will be negated once steady state has been attained. However, the possibility of adverse interactions between highly protein-bound drugs should be remembered.

e. Drug distribution

Changes in lean body mass and fat mass as well as body water lead to changes in drug distribution with age. As a result, lipid-soluble drugs will have a larger distribution volume (V_d) and therefore lower plasma level, while polar drugs have a small V_d and a high plasma level.

f. End-organ sensitivity

Considerable evidence exists that end-organ sensitivity increases with age, and this seems particularly to affect the nervous system. However, this may not apply to all end-organs and more research is needed in this field.

g. Excretion

Glomerular filtration rate diminishes because of reduced renal blood-flow as well as reduction in the number of glomeruli. Tubular reabsorption is altered and the sum effect is that drugs are less well excreted, as indeed are other waste products. Consequently, drug half-life is prolonged in the case of drugs dependent on renal excretion for the elimination of themselves and their metabolites.

As a result of these changes, care needs to be taken with regard to the prescription of drugs, and doses should be adjusted to meet the needs of elderly patients. The prescriber must know the pharmacology of the drug he is prescribing. He must know whether it is metabolised in the liver or excreted unchanged in the kidney.

He must know the fate and activity of its metabolites. He must know whether it is an acid or a base, whether it is highly protein-bound, whether it is lipid-soluble, and whether it is likely to interact with other drugs that the patient needs to take or is already taking.

The prescription of drugs and the management of illness in the elderly poses problems that may be more difficult to solve than they are in the younger patient who has greater reserves and resilience and therefore greater margins of safety (Royal College of Physicians Report 1984).

REFERENCES

Abrams, Joyce, Andrews K. (1984). The influence of hospital admission on long term medication of elderly patients. *J. Roy. Coll. Phys. Lond.*; **18**: 225–7.

Bird T., Hall M. R. P., Schade R. O. K. (1977). Gastric histology and its relation to anaemia in the elderly. *Gerontology*; **23**: 309–21.

Blichert-Toft M. (1975). Secretion of corticotrophin and somatotrophin by the senescent adrenohypophysis in man. *Acta Endocrin., Copnh, Suppl.*; **195**.

Bunker, Valda W., Lawson, Margaret S., Delves H. T., and Clayton, Barbara (1982). Metabolic balance studies for zinc and nitrogen in healthy elderly subjects. *Human Nutrition: Clinical Nutrition*; **36C**: 213–21.

Bunker, Valda W., Lawson, Margaret S., Delves H. T. and Clayton, Barbara (1984). The intake and excretion of lead and cadmium by the elderly. *Am. J. Clin. Nutr.*; **39**. 803–8.

Bunker Valda W., Lawson, Margaret S., Delves H. T. and Clayton, Barbara (1984). The uptake and excretion of chromium by the elderly. *Am. J. Clin. Nutr.*; **39**: 797–802.

Caird F. I. (1980). Editorial, *J. Clin. Exp. Gerontol.*; **2**: III-IV.

Cartlidge N. E. F., Black M. M., Hall M. R. P., Hall R. (1970). Pituitary function in the elderly. *Geront. Clin.*; **12**: 65–70.

Department of Health and Social Security (1972). *A nutrition survey of the elderly. Report on Public Health and Social Subjects, No. 3*. London: HMSO.

Department of Health and Social Security (1979). *Nutrition and health in old age. Report on Health and Social Subjects, No. 16*. London: HMSO.

Exton-Smith A. N. (1980). Nutritional Status: Diagnosis and prevention of malnutrition. In *Metabolic and Nutritional Disorders in the Elderly* (Exton-Smith A. N., Caird F. I. eds.) pp. 66–76. Bristol: John Wright & Sons.

Jeffreys P. M. (1972). The prevalence of thyroid disease in patients admitted to a geriatric department. *Age & Ageing*; **1**: 33–7.

Judge T. G. (1980). Potassium and Magnesium. In *Metabolic and Nutritional Disorders in the Elderly* (Exton-Smith, A. N., Caird F. I., eds.) pp. 39–44. Bristol: John Wright & Sons.

Lutwak L., Krook L., Henriksson T. A. et al. (1971). Calcium deficiency and human periodontal disease. *Isr. J. Med. Sci.*; **7**: 504–5.

MacLennan W. J., Martin P., Mason B. J. (1975). Causes for reduced dietary intake in a long-stay hospital. *Age & Ageing*; **4**: 175–80.

MacLeod, Catriona C. (1972). Methods of dietary assessment. In *Symposia of the Swedish Nutrition Foundation: Nutrition in old age*. (Carlson L. A. ed.), pp. 118–22.

Nilas L., Christiansen C., Rodbro P. (1984). Calcium supplementation and postmenopausal bone loss. *Br. Med. J.*; **2**: 1103–6.

Report of the Royal College of Physicians (1984). Medication for the elderly. *J. Roy. Coll. Phys. Lond.*; **18**: 7–17.

Smith M. J., Hall M. R. P. (1973). Carbohydrate tolerance in the very aged. *Diabetologia*; **9**: 387–91.

Thomas, Anita J., Briggs R. S., Monro P. (1984). Is leucocyte ascorbic acid an unreliable estimate of vitamin C deficiency? *Age & Ageing*; **13**: 243–7.

Thurnham D. (1972). Quoted by Exton-Smith A. N. *Vitamins in Metabolic and Nutritional Disorders in the Elderly*. (Exton-Smith A. N., Caird F. I., eds.) p. 29. Bristol: John Wright & Sons.

Werner I. (1983). Nutritional characteristics of the elderly. In *Geriatrics 2* (Platt D., ed.) pp. 352–65. Berlin: Springer Verlag.

Wilson T. S., Datta S. B., Murrell J. S. et al. (1973). Relation of vitamin C levels to mortality in a geriatric hospital: a study of the effect of vitamin C administration. *Age & Ageing*; **2**: 163–71.

Section II

Chapter 5

Delivery of Care

R. B. JOHNS

INTRODUCTION

The dental treatment of patients who are elderly can provide the practitioner with a challenge to his professionalism, judgement and ingenuity, as well as a test of his sense of caring for the well-being of the community in which he lives. For those who accept the challenge the rewards are varied, stimulating and often surprising.

Broadly speaking the delivery of dental care is seen as being either in the surgery or in the place where the patient lives. It is, however, important to keep in mind that this division should not be regarded as inflexible. Indeed, it is likely that many patients will progress from the former to the latter and sometimes back again, depending on home circumstances and on the type of treatment to be provided. Home care should be a part of the dentist's obligation to those who seek his professional services, whatever their age.

In this chapter these two particular aspects, treatment in the surgery and away from it, will be considered separately. It is important, however, to be aware of a period of change from one to the other.

FACILITIES FOR PATIENTS ATTENDING FOR TREATMENT

The exterior

The design of premises for a practice should from the outset take into account the special needs of a whole range of patients who will attend. This applies not only to the elderly and to the very young but also to all those who are physically or mentally handicapped.

The entrance to a practice or a hospital department should provide easy access from a car and, if possible, there should be car parking facilities near at hand. It is certainly worth establishing an entrance that will allow a wheelchair to be brought into the premises, if not into the surgery itself. If this is not possible and the chair has to be left outside, then it must be kept both safe and dry.

The interior

If access from the street or the interior design of the premises involves stairs, or even only two or three steps, then a hand-rail should always be provided. Good lighting and a non-slip floor covering are also an essential part of any design of premises which those with impaired sight or balance may be expected to use.

Ideally, the waiting room should include the following features: provision for those who have difficulty in rising after being seated for a while; sturdy chairs with strong arm rests; good lighting and non-slip floor covering; and the avoidance of hazards in the form of low tables. In addition, favourable siting and design of toilet facilities is desirable, with particular attention to the provision of hand-rails.

Finally, if at all possible, a small room or area apart from the main thoroughfare of the practice or hospital department should be available after treatment for repairing make-up and adjusting hair, and for patients to compose themselves.

Staff

Ancillary staff, particularly those responsible for the reception of patients, must be made especially aware of the needs of the elderly. The journey from the waiting room to the surgery may take more time for an elderly person and allowance should be made for this when the dentist is ready to see the patient. The hazards *en route* should of course be reduced to a minimum.

It is important that the receptionist and the dental nurse are both clear in their speech and ready to offer an arm or a hand to help, particularly to a new patient unfamiliar with both the environment and those being met for the first time. It is the dental nurse who is the link in the introduction of the new patient to the dentist and the conventions of such introductions should always be observed. The small amount of extra time taken to ensure the polite formalities, particularly for those who may be apprehensive and marginally confused, is a small investment for the benefits of establishing a good professional rapport with a new patient from the outset.

The consultation

The busy or rushed dentist should never lose sight of the fact that the visit by an elderly patient may well have taken much planning and it is likely that friends or relations have also become involved in the logistics of the visit. Although this has already been stated in Chapter 1, it is worth emphasising that, for the patient, the visit may well be the event of the week. Punctuality in keeping an appointment is often keenly noted by patients in these circumstances. No hint of being in a rush himself should be given by the dentist at this or any other time. Once the introductions are over the initial questions should be posed in a calm and methodical manner. These may be either with the patient seated in an upright position in the dental chair or preferably, if facilities are available, at a desk remote from the dental chair. Whichever is decided upon it is particularly important for the patient to have a chance to acclimatise to the surroundings and to the voice of the dentist and to be able to see his face while talking. This can help the patient to understand the questions and can indicate to the dentist the correct rate at which his questions should be delivered.

The importance of making good records is paramount. The skill to sift that which is relevant from the trivia can test even the most experienced. However, the trivia are sometimes worthy of note as they can give the patient a sense of being well cared for when such items are referred to at subsequent visits. The record card should also indicate any special facilities the particular patient may need. Medication that the patient is currently receiving or has received of late must be noted and a brief request for verification of these facts from the patient's medical practitioner is a wise precaution.

The dental chair

Access to the dental chair should be uncluttered to allow for the use of a walking stick or even a Zimmer frame. A supporting arm from the dentist or dental nurse should be offered with tact as it may be regarded as an affront to the patient's independence and be rebuffed peremptorily.

The dental chair itself should be adjusted to a sitting position and be at an appropriate height for the patient's stature. If there is an arm-rest on the side of entry, it is sometimes better to remove this or place it out of the way until the patient is seated. The provision of an arm-rest on both sides is undoubtedly of help to patients who are overweight or have weakness in their back muscles.

Seated or supine?

It is important to discuss the question of the most appropriate position for the chair with the patient. Many patients grew up in the era when they sat upright for all dental treatment. Any but the slightest change from this position may be regarded with suspicion and distrust. For patients with breathing problems or those who are obese, the tipping back of a chair can cause alarm and respiratory embarrassment. It shows courtesy on the part of the dentist if he defers to the preference of the patient who, once a degree of trust has been established, may well agree to or even request treatment in the supine position. It is facts such as these which need to be noted carefully on the record card.

When adjustments are made to a headrest or during the period of clinical examination it is wise to note if a wig or hairpiece is worn by the patient. Displacement of items of this nature can cause acute embarrassment, so that even reference to their existence is better avoided; again it is wise merely to note the fact on the record card.

The examination

Unless there has been a necessity to attend to an acute dental condition, the first visit is better confined to the establishment of an understanding of the problems posed. A thorough clinical and, if necessary, radiographic examination as well as a medical and dental history must be recorded. If the treatment required is straightforward this can be outlined immediately, with the patient sitting upright in the chair and the dentist sitting in a direct line of vision. Alternatively the treatment can be discussed at a desk with or without a friend or relation being present. Words and phrases should be carefully chosen and delivered in a manner that will ensure their being understood and again this period of explanation should not be hurried. Time and an invitation to the patient to ask questions must also be allowed. Undoubtedly the presence of a friend or relative not only helps to ensure that what has been said is understood, but it provides an instant second opinion for the patient who may be a little bewildered.

A sensitivity to the patient's awareness of being elderly is of first importance at this time, as has already been pointed out in Chapter 1. Any indication of being patronising or talking about the patient in the third person is to be avoided if a proper rapport is to be established. It is certainly inappropriate to indulge in the kind of phrase that implies: 'Well, it is only to be expected at your age.' It should also be appreciated that elderly patients do have their 'off'days; an abrupt manner at one visit may merely be a sign of one such day.

Being considerate

It is not intended in a chapter devoted to the delivery of care to enter into details of operative techniques that may be employed. These are covered in Chapters 6 and 7. It is perhaps appropriate, however, to stress the extra care necessary when treating the elderly. It must not be forgotten that all the tissues of the mouth and face become increasingly fragile with age. Susceptibility to bruising requires special mention: for example, if the extraction of a lower tooth is necessary, care must be taken to protect the skin overlying the mandible from excessive concentration of pressure from fingers or thumb supporting the jaw. Similarly, cotton wool rolls which do not become saturated with saliva or water spray need to be moistened before their removal from the mouth in order to avoid damage to the mucous membrane.

Eye protection is important, and tinted spectacles may be more comfortable for the patient in a brightly-lit surgery. It is better to avoid those that are too dark, however, since eye contact between the patient and the dentist or the dental nurse is an important facet of communication. When giving a patient protective spectacles of this nature, it must again be remembered that the patient may be wearing a wig and deference to this is necessary.

Self care

Oral hygiene, although perhaps adequately performed for many years, can suddenly deteriorate as a result of some minor physical disability such as a strained arm or wrist. Alternatively the patient may have suffered a stroke which has completely destroyed the ability to clean his teeth. It is commonplace to find that chronic arthritis has made oral hygiene procedures progressively more difficult. When conditions of this nature have impaired ability to clean the teeth, the use of an electric toothbrush may be necessary. The construction of a simple device to enlarge the handle of a normal brush may, however, suffice to solve the difficulty.

It is noticeable that the elderly often appear to maintain a plateau as regards their physical and mental abilities. Deterioration of either or both states then seems to occur suddenly as a consequence of some apparently minor episode. However, sudden bereavement often leads to a generalised lack of care that manifests itself in ways other than a lack of oral care.

DOMICILIARY VISITS

In Britain, most elderly people live either on their own or with relatives; of the rest, a small number live in warden-supervised housing but most live in old people's homes and long-stay geriatric hospitals. Unless regular dental care has been a normal part of their lives it is all too easy for routine dental inspection to be overlooked by the elderly themselves or by those who take care of them. As with chiropody, treatment is usually sought only as a result of pain and discomfort. A fractured denture, a jagged tooth or a long-standing ulcer that will not heal are among the more common complaints.

It is important to enable those who care for the elderly, whether relatives, wardens or matrons, to be made aware that there are dentists who will attend to the dental needs of the elderly on a domiciliary basis. The initial contact with an Old People's Home usually results from some minor dental emergency. The warden or matron telephones every dental practice in the area until a sympathetic reply is received. The staff of a home, health visitor or general medical practitioner are sometimes forthcoming about the dental problems of those in their care when they themselves are receiving dental treatment. This is certainly an occasion when the service of the dentist can quite properly be proffered, though care and tact are required at all levels when offering to provide dental treatment for new patients, lest a charge of advertising is incurred. Practitioners unwilling to provide such a service themselves are sometimes extremely vigilant in this respect.

Patients in geriatric wards are in the charge of a consultant who will, in most instances, be able to call upon the services of a dental colleague. However, a patient who has regularly attended a dental practice for many years may indicate a wish to be seen by his own dentist. At the request of the consultant in charge of the patient, it is possible to arrange for the patient's own dentist to attend to his needs. Care must, of course, be taken to inform all those within the hospital administration of the consultant's agreement and that of his dental colleagues. Other formalities may be requested by the hospital authorities before treatment can be provided.

Visit to patient's home

It is those patients who attend a dental practice on a regular basis, be they relative, neighbour or home help, who usually form the link between the dentist and the housebound patient with a dental problem. In common with many initial consultations, it is the so-called 'emergency' that establishes this contact. The manner and alacrity with which the episode is handled by the dentist is often the major criterion on which he is judged. For this reason, it is wise to have an 'emergency' kit to hand so that a quick response is possible. The fact that the problem may have been predictable or even present for some time is no reason for delaying a response when help is requested.

The question of the financial basis on which the visit is to be made, either immediately or for any long-term arrangement, is a matter for a clear statement by the dentist, with due regard to professional obligation and integrity. The patient and those associated with the patient, whether friends, relatives or neighbours, should be left in no doubt about such arrangements; the basis upon which the treatment is being provided and will be provided in the future must be made clear.

Whatever preconceived views have been formed about a patient when seen at the practice, it often comes as a revelation to see him in his own surroundings. Home visiting is rarely a part of the education of a dental student and it must be kept constantly in mind, particularly by those new to this experience, that one is a guest in the home. In spite of this, however, it should be appreciated at the same time that one is going to be expected to take charge. It is a situation which is commonplace for the medical practitioner, the health visitor and the district nurse, but for a dentist the environment is unusual and, removed from the security of his own surgery, he may well feel ill at ease.

As many elderly patients live alone it is particularly important to establish clear and unambiguous lines of communication. It is undoubtedly helpful on the first visit to have a relative, neighbour or friend of the patient present, not only to help with domestic arrangements but to listen to what is being said. The presence of a second person who can act as a counsellor, interpreter and reporter of what took place when the visit is over and being relived by the patient, is of considerable benefit.

If the so-called emergency that prompts the first visit is a matter of days rather than hours ahead, a clearly written note indicating the time and day of the visit will certainly remove some of the anxiety many old people feel when strangers are to visit them. Unannounced calling is certainly to be avoided for new patients if at all possible. An immediate response to an emergency will not cause such constraints.

The necessity to have a relative or friend in attendance at subsequent visits will have to be judged on the type of treatment envisaged, as well as on the physical and mental robustness of the patient. It is better to err on the side of having someone else about – or at least in the house – if in any doubt. The value of a second witness to any advice or directions given to the patient is of undoubted benefit and may need to be supplemented with clearly written instructions.

It is well to remember that many people who live on their own have 'call codes', such as a particular sequence of doorbell rings, which the practitioner may be invited to use. These simple security precautions will need to be noted on the record cards not only to facilitate the answering of the door but also to help establish a rapport with the patient.

Conditions within the house vary enormously and must be taken into account when assessing the patient; the medical history and the reported dental problems must also take account of these conditions. It is wise to note on the record card all those items not available or not of a standard considered acceptable. If the patient is bedridden, severe limitations on treatment are imposed. Nevertheless such patients have usually established the use of numerous pillows which support their body in a sitting-up position. With a little ingenuity some form of head support is possible, although at times one may have to resort to the use of hand support by a dental nurse.

The improvised dental chair

When a patient is able to sit in a chair, good access around it is important. High-backed chairs, especially those with wings, can present considerable difficulties. A firm semi-upholstered chair, to which a simple form of headrest may be attached, is probably the best compromise that can be reached. Tall dentists or those with back problems must be particularly wary of accepting a patient in a position which will cause undesirable strain in their own posture. If, on the initial assessment and examination visit, no suitable chair can be found then it may be necessary for the dentist to bring one of his own. A wheelchair, although expensive, is not only easier to transport but is also easier to adapt with regard to a headrest and even minor tilting.

The improvised surgery

The choice of room will often depend on the mobility of the patient but may also rest on the ease and access round the chair once the patient is seated. The kitchen is likely to be the most suitable room but the living room may have to suffice if that is the one chosen by the patient. Sensitivity to the patient's wishes is most important and, although the dentist is 'in charge', it is probably unwise to impose one's own views too strongly and so initiate unnecessary conflict.

Great care must, of course, be taken to protect work surfaces offered by the patient, so that a set of suitable mats, as well as paper or plastic table cloths, should be taken on all visits. Treasured items of furniture and floor coverings which seem to be ordinary and commonplace may well be held in high regard by the patient and therefore must be protected and respected accordingly.

Before leaving

When treatment is completed it is for both the dentist and the dental nurse to ensure that all is as it was before the visit and that all waste and rubbish is collected and taken away. Before leaving it is necessary to ensure that the patient, and whoever else was present, is made well aware of the treatment that has been carried out and any likely consequences. This must be expressed in appropriate terms which are understood by those involved. Any instructions concerning after-care, as well as the date and time of the next visit, should be spoken as well as written. Distinct writing with a dark felt pen is a wise precaution to avoid misunderstandings. Again it is important to give unambiguous instructions concerning methods of obtaining advice or help should these be required over a weekend or public holiday.

Care must be taken with subsequent appointments to avoid conflict with other services or visitors expected by the patient. The list of those who call can sometimes seem endless, including the chiropodist, the hairdresser, the district nurse, the health visitor, the meals on wheels service – to say nothing of the doctor and visits to the hospital. There is, it sometimes appears, a contradiction to the loneliness which is claimed by some old people.

VISITS TO OLD PEOPLE'S HOMES

Once a contact with an Old People's Home has been established, and it is seen that more than a simple denture repair service is required, a visit to the Home and an interview with the Matron or Warden should be made. At this visit the extent of the service that can be provided should be outlined and an idea obtained of the likely requests from the residents for dental treatment. It is important to know whether any other practitioners visit the patients in the Home in order to avoid any possible embarrassment this could cause. Professional courtesies should be observed and some cooperation may usefully be established.

The facilities which the Home can provide will be variable, but a so-called sickroom or treatment room is usually to be found. It may well be that it is the same room as the one used when the doctor, the chiropodist or the hairdresser visits, and booking of the room may be necessary.

The importance of establishing a good rapport with both the Matron and the staff cannot be overstated. Both can be a most useful source of general information about the residents but, although the medical history and drug regime may be obtained from within the Home, it is wise to verify this with the medical practitioner who attends the Home if the history should appear at all complex.

The mental alertness of the patient needs careful assessment. Seemingly quite rational residents who are remarkably adept at sustaining an illusion over a short period can give bizarre histories. A responsible member of the staff certainly needs to be on hand at the time of the initial assessment.

Not only does this impart a sense of security for a patient who, to a greater or lesser extent, is 'institutionalised' but the accuracy of the information given by the patient can easily be verified. Moreover, if some decisions have to be made, then the patient can seek advice from a person familiar to him and, at the same time, there will be a reliable witness to what has been said and what has taken place.

Patients who live in Old People's Homes inevitably tend to be less self-reliant than their counterparts living alone. A visit to a dental surgery, although physically possible for many of those patients who live in a Home, can easily engender unnecessary anxiety. The mere thought of being called upon to deal with the outside world once more is too disturbing. This feeling is then grafted on to the anxiety about the dental problem to be faced and together they can exacerbate the problems of the dental treatment out of all proportion. However, it is necessary to be aware of the reverse reaction, namely that some of the residents may well be mentally alert and independent and may welcome a reason to justify an excursion out of the Home and back to the outside world. These patients can easily be affronted if dealt with in a similar manner to their more timorous and 'institutionalised' fellow residents.

The room which is to be made available should be inspected and careful note made of those services that are and are not provided. When several Homes are visited, such information should be readily available to the ancillary staff in the practice who prepare equipment to be taken on a visit (see check list, p. 136). In common with most institutions, there is usually a routine within a Home, and it is important to be aware of such arrangements. The extent of this routine is not confined to meal times; regular visits by numerous individuals and organisations should be noted and avoided if possible.

Warden-controlled flats or apartments

Those who live in this form of accommodation are in an environment halfway between living alone and living in an Old People's Home. There is usually a warden nearby who may be regarded in much the same way as the Matron of a Home and from whom much background information may be obtained. It is also necessary to ensure that he or she is provided with all the information pertinent to any dental treatment which has been carried out.

The dental nurse

The role of the dental nurse is extremely important in the organisation and delivery of domiciliary dental care, including the careful making of appointments as well as notes and instructions, and the organisation of the clinical work. A good knowledge of the neighbourhood is needed in order to plan what might be a number of visits in the most appropriate sequence. Her responsibilities in preparing the equipment and materials required for the treatment of, possibly, numerous patients at several different sites are considerable. Laboratory work appropriate to each patient must be taken in clearly labelled containers. If impressions are to be cast during the period away from the surgery then all necessary materials and equipment should be included in the domiciliary kit.

Besides being adaptable and being able to improvise normal surgery routines, sometimes at very short notice, the nurse must be particularly sensitive to the needs of the patient. The environment and conditions for work will on occasion test the ingenuity of both the dentist and the nurse alike, and each must be aware of the other's problems. It is above all the freshness and enthusiasm which the dental nurse can bring to such visits that the elderly find appealing.

Hospitality

Sensitivity to the offer of hospitality by patients is essential. It is as well to be prepared either for a small gift at the end of a course of treatment or for a cup of tea as a mark of gratitude at the end of a visit. Refusal of either can be interpreted as an affront.

The range of hospitality and the dentist's involvement in it can be considerable. There are undoubtedly some patients who get much pleasure from engineering a meeting between those who represent different facets of their life. The introduction of grown up children or grandchildren is important to them and this should be recognised as the compliment it is. Neither should it be forgotten that the dentist and his nurse may represent the 'breath of fresh air' from the world outside for which many of the elderly may crave, particularly if they have no close family who call on them.

The glimpses of and involvement in other lives is not only interesting and sometimes educational but nearly always rewarding. It is without doubt one of the major benefits of undertaking domiciliary dentistry.

Equipment

The range of equipment necessary for a domiciliary visit will usually require the use of a car. Although it may not be necessary to take much in the way of equipment into a patient's home, it is wise to have additional items readily available for unforeseen contingencies. It is important to make the car secure when parked outside a patient's home, and also to ensure that items of equipment left in the car cannot be easily seen by the casual observer who may easily turn into the petty pilferer.

The collection of equipment, under various categories, into boxes or cases that can easily be carried is important. These items should themselves be clearly identifiable in order to make their checking, both out of the surgery and into the car at the end of a visit, less vulnerable to error.

It is also better to have individual items that can easily be carried by one person and to bear in mind the situations through which the equipment may need to pass. Damage to paintwork or furniture from the sharp corners of boxes or cases can be inflicted all too easily and every effort should be made to minimise such a risk. Besides being thoughtless and impolite, causing damage of this nature is likely to give a poor impression to all concerned.

The range of treatment intended will obviously determine the equipment and materials necessary for such visits. If it is intended to make domiciliary dentistry a significant aspect of the practice then it may be felt justifiable to equip the equivalent of a whole dental surgery in transportable form. However it is more likely that the equipment will be built up in stages in the light of experience of the demand encountered. Initially, besides a number of simple examination kits and appropriate record cards, the items necessary for simple extractions, inserting sutures, and placing dressings in teeth, are all that is required. This range of equipment and materials may soon need supplementing with items that allow the dentist to deal with the relining or construction of complete dentures (see Chapter 7). Most of the items used will have to be taken out of general use within the surgery. For this reason it is important to prepare lists of items required and, indeed, to mark all such instruments and perhaps even materials to assist in their collection. Irritating oversights may thus be avoided.

Although plastic tool-kit boxes are often suitable for some equipment, particularly that associated with denture construction, a better impression is created by the use of various proprietary boxes, such as 'cool boxes', or those designed to take the numerous items necessary to accompany babies and small children. These can readily be adapted for dental use.

Expensive transportable equipment is now available and provides all those facilities that can be expected in a well-equipped surgery. These include the 'conventional' and 'ultra-high-speed' air turbine handpieces, ultrasonic scaler, three-in-one syringe, high-vacuum suction, an operating light, a capsule-mixing facility, fibre-optic composite-curing light, head lamp attachment and x-ray film viewing screen. Equipment of this nature will, however, represent a large capital expenditure which, unless it is shared, must inevitably remain under-used in most circumstances.

The sample check lists that follow should only be regarded as a general indication of what is required and in no way comprise an exclusive list. Individual variations are, after all, the spice of clinical dentistry.

APPENDIX – CHECK LIST

Examination kit

Equipment	Materials
Pen torch light	Cotton wool rolls
Lighted mouth mirror	Gauze squares
Mouth mirrors	Medical paper tissues
Probes	Ethyl chloride
Tweezers	Temporary filling material

Instruments for manipulating
temporary filling material
Clip-on light
Electric adaptors
Electric tumbler heater
Multi-outlet extension lead
Chip syringe
Plastic bowl to act as spittoon
Magnifying loupes

Protective spectacles
Hand mirror
Bib
Model-maker electric motor
capable of taking dental burs

Surface disinfectant

Mouth wash
Plastic tumblers
Plastic denture bowls
Paper towels
Hand-washing materials
Rubber gloves
Denture marking equipment
(for use in geriatric wards
and Old People's Homes)
Plastic bags for waste, and
sealing device

Prosthetic kit for complete dentures

It is assumed that all those items suggested in the Examination kit
and Administrative kit (see p. 138) would also be available.

Equipment

Mixing bowl
Spatula
Measures for impression
materials when indicated
Selection of impression trays
Shade/mould guide
Wax knife
Spirit lamp
Mat for spirit lamp (wax-
proof)
Ruler
Bite gauge
Portable electric drill/
handpiece
Stones/trimming burs
Denture duplicating kit
Wax block trimming device
File

Laboratory work as appropriate

Materials

Impression materials
Mixing pads
Plastic bags which can be
sealed
Waxes
Matches/lighter
Adhesive for trays
Indelible pencil
Sandpaper

Articulating paper
Denture-cleaning materials
Pressure-detecting paste
Ointment for ulcers
Disclosing tablets
Lubricating jelly

If any electrical equipment is to be used, it is wise to test the polarity of the socket and the effectiveness of the insulated covering of the equipment. If in any doubt consult a qualified electrician. Equipment using rechargeable batteries is both safer and more versatile.

Surgical equipment

Many items are currently available in a sterile prepacked form, and these are of considerable value when surgical treatment is required in the domestic environment.

Items, such as extraction forceps, that need to be sterile should either be transported after sterilisation in an appropriately packaged container or in an unopened domestic pressure cooker which has been through a sterilising cycle. Small items that will not be damaged by the higher temperatures of a glass bead steriliser may be treated in such a device. This item may, indeed, be taken on visits as it will allow re-sterilisation of small instruments in the event of inadvertent contamination.

Administrative kit

Record cards, additional card for special requirements
Local map
Appointment cards
Instruction cards/emergency instructions, printed or
  pre-written
Broad felt pen
Appointment book
Laboratory instruction book (duplicate)
Notebook to record special requirements
A day-book
Prescription pad
Prescriber's formulary

IMPLICATIONS FOR DENTAL EDUCATION

Justification for inclusion in undergraduate course

At the present time there are more than 9.5 million people of pensionable age in Britain, i.e. approximately 17% of the population. It is considered that this proportion will increase only slightly by the end of the century. However, the actual number of over-75s in the population is predicted to rise from 3.1 million in 1978 to 4.2 million, and over-85s from just above half a million in 1978 to 1.1 million, by the year 2000. From these figures it is clear that all health services need to prepare themselves now for a marked increase in the demands of the elderly.

To some extent, the dental problems of this group have in the past been overlooked by many dentists who have regarded the demands of young people as more urgent and more deserving of their services. Moreover the structure of fees within the National Health Service has provided little financial inducement for practitioners to seek out work with the elderly unless strongly motivated by a sense of service.

This pattern is now changing. Not only are the expectations of the population concerning dental care increasing but so is the complexity of the problems posed. Treatment of the so-called 'worn out' dentition is a particular example of the increasing dilemma which faces the dental profession.

For these reasons, as well as the decline in the restorative demands of the younger age groups and an increase in social awareness, it is now of the utmost importance that undergraduate students should have their education enhanced by courses which prepare them for this changing pattern of need.

A syllabus for undergraduates

No curriculum committee will welcome a request for additional time to be found for a new subject: it has been said that Heads of Department are like vultures all wanting their pick at the student body. It is for the Dean, or a curriculum committee, to ensure that a balanced course is maintained in the light of current understanding of the needs of dental education.

An immediate rebuttal of any request for more time in the curriculum is to be expected, often in the form of a suggestion that the new topic is better taught at a postgraduate level. Although such an approach may be justifiable for esoteric forms of treatment requiring extra teaching time, it must be unacceptable if the dental profession is to deal adequately with a problem which is gathering in momentum. By the same token, it is unrealistic to delay the introduction of a course of this nature by waiting for the whole dental course to be extended. Time must be found in the final year, or perhaps the final 18 months, to introduce lectures and seminars as well as practical experience in the field. A course of this nature, with its social and educational benefits, can only enrich the preparation of the dental student for work in the community; its interdisciplinary nature should allow all departments to forego a portion of their share in the students' timetable.

The lecture course should cover the following topics:

1. The extent of the problem posed to the community as a whole by the handicapped and the elderly, in terms of their general needs as well as those specific to dentistry.
2. The role the dentist has to play in meeting the needs of those in the community who are unable to attend a hospital, health centre or surgery without recourse to ambulance services.
3. The ageing processes and their effect on the oral tissues.
4. The psychology of ageing and the psychology of dealing with the elderly.
5. The techniques associated with the delivery of dental care to the elderly.

It is also important that students should be exposed to the problems of working away from a fully equipped surgery. This experience should be seen as a normal part of general practice and therefore should be based on the General Practice Unit which is part of the school. By virtue of the close supervision and teaching necessary for domiciliary dental care, the member of staff responsible should form an integral part of the Unit.

The organisation of extramural visits for undergraduates

Although visits to a full variety of the places where a dentist may be called upon to provide dental care for the elderly or handicapped would be difficult to arrange, at least a representative sample should be included in the extramural programme. The problems associated with each sample would clearly form a basis for information discussed and students should be encouraged not only to point out difficulties they see but also to proffer their own solutions.

In addition to organised visits to see a variety of establishments and perhaps observe members of the staff providing treatment for patients, it is important that students themselves have opportunities to undertake some clinical work. Once a means of identifying those patients who are in need of straightforward treatment in their own home has been established then one or two students, accompanied by a member of the teaching staff, should if possible see the treatment through to completion.

Voluntary work by students in Old People's Homes or Geriatric Wards should also be encouraged, so that a general understanding of the problems of caring for the elderly can be engendered.

The identification of those in need of dental care

The identification of those who are in need of dental care within their own home is often seen as a difficulty in a teaching hospital. Careful scrutiny of a waiting list, and the following up of patients who fail to attend after assessment but before treatment has started, provides an initial list. It is also possible to offer the service to those patients who are seen to be having difficulty in attending regularly. The mere fact of providing a service of this nature will of itself generate, by word of mouth, an increase in demand.

Direct contact with the whole range of support services now available, organised both by the local health authority and by private organisations, will undoubtedly widen the knowledge of what is possible in respect of domiciliary dental care.

The information can be further disseminated by informing local medical and dental practitioners as well as the Senior Dental Officer for the District. It is clear that cooperation with local dental practitioners and the Community Dental Service is of the utmost importance.

It is important to inform all those within the dental hospital and school of the initiation of such a service. It is equally important that consultant geriatricians in nearby hospitals are made aware of the introduction of this facet of dental education.

The experience of students may be further increased if local dental practitioners, who themselves provide domiciliary care, are prepared to take one or two students with them on their visits. Arrangements of this nature obviously demand careful organisation on the part of the member of staff in the General Practice Unit in charge of domiciliary care.

Chapter 6

Restorative Needs and Methods

R. J. IBBETSON

INTRODUCTION

It is the purpose of this chapter to consider the restorative management of elderly patients. There is no possibility that this discussion can cover all aspects of tooth restoration. The aim, therefore, is to deal with areas of prime importance in the treatment of the elderly, and particularly with conditions which may be different from those seen in most adult patients. An attempt will also be made to cover topics of importance which are often absent from text-books on restorative dentistry. The restorative needs of the elderly are determined by the patterns of dental disease affecting them, but more than in any other age group it may be necessary to adapt treatment to suit the individual. This need for compromise is not something that can be easily determined; nevertheless, it must be remembered that restorative dentistry is carried out for the benefit of the patient rather than the operator.

There are indications that one of the strongest influences on the type of treatment provided for the elderly is the attitude of the dentist to such patients. The tendency exists to see the elderly as poor candidates for restorative work. In addition, many of these individuals are likely to believe that ill-health and disability are inevitable. The combination of these approaches may preclude the patient from seeking, or the dentist from providing, the necessary restorative care. The general restorative needs of the elderly patient are no different from those of other age groups. These may be summarised as the maintenance of comfort, aesthetics and function. These needs must be balanced against the ability of the elderly to receive treatment; the latter may be influenced by the patients' state of health, whether they are ambulatory, and their tolerance of dental procedures.

Pattern of disease

Dental status will be greatly influenced by previous patterns of dental disease and by treatment which patients have received earlier in life. In addition, the age changes of the teeth and surrounding structures make a marked contribution to the problems confronting the restorative dentist. Whilst it is impossible to determine the precise contribution that each of these factors makes, they combine to produce the clinical conditions commonly seen in the elderly patient. It is reasonable to assume that many elderly patients will have lost one or more teeth from the effects of dental disease experienced over many years. The replacement of all missing teeth is not necessarily indicated; it must be considered, however, either on aesthetic grounds or when loss of teeth interferes with the patient's ability to function satisfactorily. Not surprisingly, in view of the length of time for which the teeth have been functional, the effects of wear may be observed on the occlusal, facial and/or lingual surfaces of the teeth. The aetiology varies in complexity and careful diagnosis is necessary if restorative management of the patient is to be successful.

A common feature of teeth in the elderly is an increase in length of the clinical crowns as a consequence of long-standing periodontal disease and gingival recession. This increase in the crown:root ratio may contribute to undue mobility of the teeth, whilst the exposure of areas of the root surface complicates oral hygiene procedures and renders the roots of the teeth susceptible to caries. It is a common clinical observation that the pattern of dental caries changes in the elderly. Carious lesions developing *de novo* on the surfaces of the anatomical crown are relatively uncommon. Most frequently the carious process occurs as either recurrent decay related to existing restorations or as new lesions on the root surfaces of the teeth. Indeed, root caries constitutes one of the major problems in the restorative management of elderly patients.

The combined effects of age changes within the dental tissues and previous restorative treatment may present two further problems. It has been established that restorations, particularly if placed intracoronally, tend to weaken teeth. In the older patient, these may combine with age changes within the dentine, rendering the teeth more liable to cracks and fractures. In addition, age changes within the dental pulp reduce the vitality of this tissue. It is also known that the effects of restorative procedures on the dental pulp are cumulative. These factors contribute to an increased incidence of pulp pathoses in the elderly.

THE PREVENTION OF DENTAL DISEASE

Our understanding of the nature of dental caries and periodontal disease is by no means complete. In the majority of adult patients, it may be considered that dietary control coupled with good oral hygiene procedures will minimise the incidence of both these forms of dental disease.

With this basis for the management and prevention of dental disease, it is important to remember that restorative procedures will do nothing to prevent either dental caries or periodontal disease. The only functions of restorations are to replace diseased or missing tooth structure and in some instances to protect the remaining dental hard tissues from fracture. This approach to the management of dental disease has had a great influence on the treatment of both children and adults, but its implementation in the management of the elderly patient is of the greatest importance.

In addition to the role of diet in dental caries, it is known that saliva plays an important part in preventing the disease process. One of the changes commonly occurring in the elderly patient is a reduction in salivary flow; this has obvious implications for the dental caries incidence among these individuals (see p. 77). Dietary control may be a problem for the elderly patient. Many people in this age group may live on their own and, leaving aside additional problems of concurrent medical conditions or physical disabilities, may simply not be bothered to ensure that they receive a well-balanced diet. This very often leads to a high intake of processed or pre-cooked foods; these so-called convenience foods are generally rich in fermentable carbohydrate and consequently are potentially or overtly cariogenic.

Oral hygiene

It is well known that plaque removal in adult patients often presents problems with regard to efficiency and motivation. In the elderly, these problems will often be found at an increased level. Loss of manual dexterity and reduction of the ability to concentrate inevitably reduce the efficiency of plaque control. In addition, many elderly individuals have dentitions which display increased clinical crown lengths. The exposure of root surfaces with their complex topography of grooves, concavities and flutes increases the difficulty of plaque removal. This is particularly true of the molar teeth when furcation areas become exposed to the oral environment; these areas are extremely difficult for even the most dexterous and motivated of patients to clean. A further difficulty may be sensitivity of the root surfaces when brushing the exposed dentine, which may discourage even the keenest of patients. All these factors combine to make the prevention of dental disease difficult for the majority of elderly patients. Added to this, many individuals in this age group see themselves as decrepit and they anticipate an increased incidence of illness and tooth loss as being inevitable. There is a tendency for dentists and ancillary staff, faced with these problems, to view the inevitability of dental disease in like manner. Whilst this may be true for some patients, it should be emphasised that much can be done to help and encourage the elderly.

Encouraging home care

Assessment, instruction and monitoring of plaque control procedures involve the same principles as for any patient but, for the elderly, these will require more time and attention to detail. The patient may be unable to hold a normal toothbrush; toothbrushes can be modified by changes to the handle, shape or size of the brush.

Many individual modifications may be devised, the only limiting factor being the imagination of the dentist or hygienist. For the patient who has difficulties with plaque control it is important for the dentist to ascertain the patient's capabilities, which requires assessment of plaque control procedures in the presence of the dentist. The use of disclosing solutions is essential to demonstrate to patients both what they can do and what they should be trying to achieve. Above all, it requires patience and encouragement on the part of the hygienist or dentist, especially when concerned with cleaning of the approximal surfaces of the teeth. It may be that the patient's dexterity will not support flossing or the use of wood points, but the use of small brushes with handles (e.g. 'Interspace' or 'Proxabrush') may be possible. It is again important here that the dentist does not view the patient as being incapable because he or she is old. The dentist should stress that the progress of dental disease is not inevitable and individuals must be encouraged to the limit of their capabilities to maintain their dentition. The encouragement and help must also be maintained at regular intervals; there is no set recall period to suit all patients, so that the dentist must adjust the frequency of these appointments to suit the individual's dental needs. There will be patients who, for one reason or another, are unable to remove plaque in a sufficiently effective manner. For such people, consideration must be given to regular professional prophylaxis at short intervals. This concept has implications for the work-load of those planning delivery of dental health care. However, research studies indicate that regular professional prophylaxis for patients at risk from dental disease is an effective method of control (Axelsson and Lindhe 1981: King et al. 1985).

Assessing susceptibility

It is important to be able to identify those patients who are at risk. With regard to periodontal disease, the usual diagnostic criteria should be coupled with an assessment of the degree of loss of attachment relative to the age of the patient. This will usually provide useful information about the present periodontal status and subsequent prognosis. Dental caries incidence may be hard to predict, particularly if illness or events in the patient's life, such as bereavement, bring about changes in attitude and diet. Nevertheless, a general guide to a patient's susceptibility to dental caries, and root caries in particular, may be gained from evidence of previous disease; it has been shown that there may be a correlation between previous coronal caries experience and later incidence of root caries. If these factors can be identified, then the frequency of recall appropriate for an individual may be determined.

In conclusion, it may be seen that the dental diseases found in the elderly are not different from those found amongst other adults. However, the control of the disease processes may be more difficult, with the major obstacles being created by the physiological changes which take place in ageing. Although total prevention is even less likely to be achieved for those who are disabled or ill, the management of each individual must be positive. The attitude of the dentist is of great importance in influencing the attitude of the patient. There must be determination to provide the best possible standard of dental care for each patient, rather than assuming that breakdown of the teeth and supporting structures is inevitable in the elderly. It should always be borne in mind that the majority of elderly patients are ambulatory and relatively fit.

DENTAL CARIES

There appears to be a correlation between a patient's age and the susceptibility of different sites on the teeth to dental caries. In young individuals the pits and fissures, and later the smooth surfaces, of the teeth are at risk. In the elderly patient, the effects of previous dental decay, subsequent restorations, and possible changes in the anatomy of the clinical crowns of the teeth may combine to present a very different picture. An examination of the number and type of restorations will give a good idea of the patient's previous caries experience and may be useful in predicting the risk of further carious attack. New enamel carious lesions are generally uncommon, unless the patient suffers some change in medical status or adopts a diet conducive to caries. Dental caries in the elderly most commonly involves root surfaces or appears as secondary caries around previous restorations.

Root surface caries

An increase in the length of the clinical crowns of the teeth exposes the root surfaces to the oral environment, and thus to the risk of carious attack. Root caries is not exclusively confined to the elderly. Any tooth with a long clinical crown becomes liable to carious attack in this area. The increased incidence of root caries in elderly patients reflects the greater number of root surfaces exposed. Lesions of root caries occur typically at the cement–enamel junction, probably because this is the area first exposed to the oral environment. With further exposure of the root surfaces of the teeth, lesions may be found at sites apical to the cement–enamel junction. Initially, root caries appears yellow to light-brown in colour, with the cementum and dentine becoming softened and with no sharply demarcated cavitation. Whilst our understanding of the carious process affecting the crowns of the teeth has improved, knowledge regarding the aetiology of root surface caries is still obscure (see also p. 131).

Prevention of root caries

The importance of dietary and plaque control has been discussed. This control is essential if root caries is to be prevented. The role of fluoride in prevention of enamel caries is well established and some consideration should be given to its use to protect against caries of the root surfaces. Cementum generally has a higher level of fluoride than other mineralised tissues. Root surfaces are reactive and, following exposure to the oral environment, more fluoride is taken up. However, whether this fluoride, which is bound in the tissues of the root surface as fluorhydroxyapatite, plays a significant role in preventing caries is doubtful. It is considered that the action of fluoride is due to its topical effect on carious lesions either at a subclinical or clinical level. There are at present no clinical studies that have recorded the effectiveness of fluoride in the management of root surface caries.

The restoration of teeth affected by root caries is difficult. It may well be possible that good plaque and dietary control, combined with topical fluorides, will affect remineralisation of early root carious lesions and may arrest more extensive active carious lesions. Arrest of root caries is indicated by a change in colour from the yellow or light brown appearance of the active lesions to a dark brown or even black appearance. Initial lesions begin in the subsurface layer of the root, and it is therefore prudent to avoid vigorous probing of suspected lesions lest irreversible damage to the root surface be caused.

The arrest of these carious lesions is highly desirable, and a suitable regime for prevention of root caries should therefore be adopted for all patients at risk. Dietary advice, and instruction in plaque control using a fluoride-containing toothpaste, may be supported by regular professional tooth cleaning: once again, the implications for dental manpower are significant. Fluoride may be applied in the dental surgery or at domiciliary visits, but this fluoride should not be in the form of acidified gels whose low pH is likely to decalcify the root surface. A more suitable choice would be a fluoride-containing varnish or an aqueous solution of sodium fluoride. Patients should be encouraged to use a fluoride-containing mouth-rinse on a regular basis: a 0.05% aqueous solution of sodium fluoride is suitable for daily use whilst if weekly use is considered more appropriate a 0.2% solution should be used.

Spread of lesions

Root caries typically appears as a superficial spreading lesion with a depth of 0.5–1.00mm, which does not endanger the pulp. It is found most commonly on the approximal and facial surfaces of the lower anterior and premolar teeth. It is worth considering why these are the teeth most often affected. It is likely that much of this information is derived from epidemiological studies of elderly patients, or of adult patients previously treated for periodontal disease. In both of the groups, there will be a high incidence of loss of the molar teeth. It is therefore important to bear in mind that any tooth with an exposed root surface is at risk. The superficial nature of root caries produces a spread of the lesions towards the approximo-buccal and approximo-lingual line angles of the teeth. It has been said that these shallow lesions do not often endanger the pulp; however, the thickness of dentine between the root surface and the pulp is very small in most teeth, so that lesions of only one millimetre in depth may well be in close proximity to pulpal tissue. This factor must be borne in mind where restorative procedures are undertaken.

Restoration of carious lesions of the root surface

The nature and sites of these carious lesions may make restorative treatment difficult. These problems can be classified under four main headings: the dental tissues; the nature of the lesions; the site of the lesions; the restorative materials available.

The dental tissues. The root surfaces consist of dentine covered by a thin layer of cementum, which may often be absent as a result of abrasion. Dentine behaves characteristically when cut; however, when preparing cavities on the anatomical crowns of the teeth, the dentist is able to finish the margins in enamel. This hard material allows relatively smooth margins to be achieved. On the root surface, the margins of cavities must be prepared in dentine or cementum. Compared with enamel, this tissue is relatively soft, and well-defined smooth margins are difficult, if not impossible, to create.

The nature of the lesions. The lesions of root caries are spreading in nature and, until advanced, lack obvious signs of cavitation. Wherever the initial site of the carious activity, decay spreads laterally, rather than gingivo-occlusally, to reach the line angles of the teeth. The slow superficial spread, coupled with the physical properties of dentine, can make it very difficult for the clinician to determine whether a cavity has been rendered caries-free. Considerable difficulty also arises from the lack of dentine available for the preparation of retentive features in these cavities. The tendency for spread to occur towards the line angles of the teeth increases the difficulty in producing mechanical undercuts. The preparation of undercuts in these areas leads to undermining and loss of margins, thus further increasing the size of the preparation.

The sites. The areas of the root most commonly involved in the carious process are the facial and approximal surfaces. Examination of clinical cases and extracted teeth clearly indicates the complicated anatomy found in these areas. For a restoration to be successful, it must not only replace missing tooth structure and provide a good marginal seal, but also conform to the anatomy of the tooth if increased problems with plaque control and recurrent caries are to be avoided. This problem is compounded in many instances by inaccessibility of the lesion; the difficulties of tooth preparation when caries is present in the furcation areas of molars or on the approximal surfaces of the roots of the teeth may be severe.

The Restorative Materials. There are three different intra-coronal materials which may be used to restore teeth affected by root caries: amalgam, composite, and glass ionomer cement.

Amalgam is an excellent restorative material, but has two main disadvantages when cavities on the roots of the teeth are considered. Firstly, it requires mechanical undercuts for retention and, secondly, if the restoration is to be of good quality, adequate condensation is essential, which may be difficult if the cavity lies in an approximal surface when there is an adjacent tooth, or where a cavity has involved the furcation area of a molar.

Composite resin. The current generation of these materials shows good clinical performance when used in Class III and Class IV cavities in the crowns of anterior teeth. In combination with acid etching of enamel, a good marginal seal can be obtained, which is important for preventing discolouration and pulp damage. Modern microfilled composites will provide, in addition, a much smoother surface than has been possible with the macrofilled resins. However, where cavities are prepared in cementum and dentine, no acid etching is possible. Thus the high coefficient of thermal expansion of these materials will allow microleakage, with its possible sequelae of marginal discolouration, pulp damage and recurrent caries. In addition, mechanical

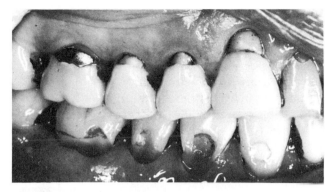

Fig 6.1 *A 60-year-old man where Class V composite restorations have been placed on root surfaces of 543. All these restorations demonstrated recurrent caries.*

retention for these restorations will be required, with all the attendant difficulties associated with creation of undercuts (Fig. 6.1).

Bonding of resin materials to dentine is still in its infancy. Advances have been made recently with the introduction of two materials – both phosphate ester/sulphonate systems – which show bonding to the mineral component of dentine. However, previous dentine-bonding agents have shown a tendency to undergo hydrolysis within the oral environment. It would seem prudent at present not to use these materials for restorations on root surfaces until adequate clinical trials have been completed.

Glass ionomer cement. This material, introduced in 1971, is a fluoride-containing ion–leachable aluminosilicate glass which is the result of a reaction between an aluminosilicate glass powder and various organic polyacids. The set material is capable of demonstrating true adhesion, via ionic and polar bonds, to both enamel and dentine, provided that the surfaces are clean.

Glass ionomer cements are thus capable of providing a good seal at the margins of a restoration placed within the root surface. Mechanical undercuts are not essential, but good resistance form is important to prevent adhesion to the tooth structure from being broken and the restoration displaced. The reaction of the dental pulp is considered to be mild. An initial acute inflammatory response soon resolves, whilst long-term studies have indicated that pulp vitality is not compromised. This material contains leachable fluoride in high concentration; it has been shown that fluoride from glass ionomer cement restorations is taken up by tooth tissue surrounding the restoration. Thus it can be anticipated that this material should provide some protection against recurrent caries.

Handling characteristics. The major problems with glass ionomer cement can arise in its handling. With any cement, the powder:liquid ratio is critical, and accurate proportioning with strict adherence to the manufacturer's instructions is critical if optimal physical properties are to be achieved. Recent developments have produced cements in which the powder containing the acid component is mixed with water; this, together with the provision of powder scoops, has reduced the difficulties of mixing.

The setting reaction of glass ionomer cement takes place in two stages. The initial set occurs within three minutes of mixing, at which stage the material may be carefully trimmed with a scalpel. The second stage is complete after seven minutes, but final maturation of the cement does not take place for at least one hour. During this time, the cement is very vulnerable to moisture contamination. To this end, the manufacturers provide resin-based varnishes for application after placement of the restoration. However, research has indicated that these varnishes are generally ineffective, and at present there appears to be no proven alternative. Current materials under test include medical grade ethyl cyanoacrylate, which is flowed as thin film from the tip of an instrument onto the restoration; alternatively, an alky-alkoxy-silane marketed as a dentine-desensitising agent (Tresiolan), has been shown to provide a relatively water-resistant film.

Restoration of a Class V carious lesion

When a carious lesion is deemed no longer amenable to treatment by attention to plaque control, diet and topical fluoride, restoration of the tooth must be undertaken. Carious lesions involving the root surface are generally close to the free gingival margin. Under such circumstances, the use of rubber dam to gain control of the operating field provides great advantages. Rubber dam application is made straightforward by isolation of at least two-thirds of one arch; with a generous number of teeth isolated, access to the area of operation is made easier. Class V cavities will generally require additional clamp placement on the tooth to be treated. In order to retract both the rubber and the gingival tissues, the use of a No. 212 Ferrier clamp is recommended for all single-rooted teeth (Fig. 6.2 (a) and (b)). For multirooted teeth an Ivory Pattern W8A usually allows good access.

Removal of caries. Carious tissue should be removed carefully, using a slowly rotating round steel bur in a contra-angle hand-piece. Following caries removal all that remains is to shape and finish the margins of the preparation to provide resistance form. This may be best carried out using a tapered or plain fissure bur, when the walls of the cavity are finished to provide a 90° cavo-surface angle. Margins should be as smooth as is practicable but it must be realised that, in dentine and cementum, they cannot be prepared to the same standard as those in enamel.

Protecting the pulp. It is recommended that, where vital dentine has been cut or the lesion is in close proximity to the pulp (which on anatomical grounds applies to virtually all root caries lesions), a protective base is applied. One of the proprietary hard-setting two-paste calcium hydroxide preparations is recommended. This should not be thicker than 0.5mm. In addition to pulp protection, this base will prevent exudation of fluid from the cut dentinal tubules – which may well interfere with both the setting reaction and adhesion of glass ionomer cement.

Use of a matrix. It is important that a matrix is used after placement of the glass ionomer cement. This will allow improved adaptation to be achieved and permit the cement to set without being disturbed. Suitable matrices are the commercially-available cervical foils, which may be readily burnished to conform to the contours of the tooth. If difficulty is experienced in holding the matrix after its initial adaptation, a convenient handle may be made by attaching the matrix to the tip of a dental hand instrument, using a small amount of molten soft ribbon wax.

Conditioning the cavity. The remaining exposed tooth tissue within the cavity is then conditioned using a 50% aqueous solution of citric acid. This does not etch the dentine, but simply provides a clean surface for the adhesion of the cement. If there is an area of unprotected prepared dentine on the floor of the cavity, the use of citric acid will cause pulp damage. Under these

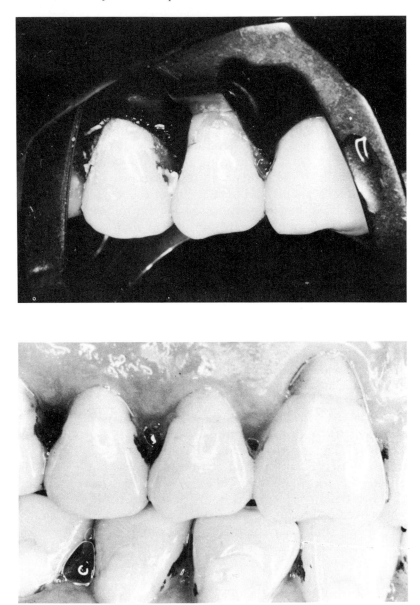

Fig 6.2   *(a) Access to Class V cavity aided by use of 212 Ferrier clamp to retract both rubber dam and gingival tissue. (b) Completed glass ionomer cement restorations 543.*

circumstances, it may be preferable to apply a solution of dilute hydrogen peroxide to the cavity to provide a clean surface, although the resultant bond between the cement and the tooth structure will be somewhat weaker.

Inserting the restoration. The cement is mixed according to the manufacturer's instructions, inserted into the cavity, and the matrix placed and held in position until the initial set is complete. On removal of the matrix, the excess cement is trimmed carefully with a sharp scalpel to clear the margins and refine the contour. The cement should be trimmed parallel to the margins of the cavity in order to avoid the risk of the cement being pulled away from the cavity walls. If further finishing is required, the cement must be allowed to complete the second stage of its setting reaction before this is carried out. Following this, gentle finishing and contouring may be carried out, using a lubricated white stone at very slow speed.

Heat generated during this procedure will damage the cement, however, and if reasonable contour has been achieved following trimming of the restoration with the scalpel, it is advisable to carry out final finishing at a subsequent appointment when the risk of damage to the restoration is less likely.

The restoration is checked for marginal integrity and contour. A protective coat of cyanoacrylate cement is applied to the restoration and allowed to dry. The rubber dam is removed, and the patient can then leave. At a subsequent visit, if further finishing is required, this may be carried out using a white stone in a contra-angle handpiece but, in order to avoid damaging the mature set cement, heat and dehydration must be avoided; consequently these final procedures must be carried out under waterspray and high speeds must be avoided.

Restoration of teeth with approximal carious lesions of the root surface where there are adjacent teeth

In posterior teeth, if root caries on an approximal surface involves an existing amalgam restoration, it may be reasonable to remove the existing restoration via an occlusal approach in order to gain access to the carious lesion. Such cavities may be very suitable for restoration with amalgam, since mechanical retention may be easily produced and straight-line access for condensation is possible. However, particular care must be taken

with matrix placement and adaptation. In all instances an approximal wedge is essential and, due to the long clinical crown, the
matrix may have to be adapted further by the use of softened
brown stick compound, which is forced into the approximal
area. On removal of the matrix, the restoration should be
examined and trimmed to ensure that the contour of the restoration conforms to that of the tooth. In cases where there is no
pre-existing restoration or where the carious lesion is
significantly separated from such a restoration, an occlusal
approach for cavity preparation would be unnecessarily destructive. In such cases, an approach from the facial or lingual aspect
should be made, creating a slot preparation.

Access. The choice between the buccal or the lingual approach is
determined by ease of access and by the site of the carious lesion
being closer to one aspect than another. Once again, the benefits
of rubber dam placement are considerable. If difficulty is encountered due to visibility being obscured by heaping-up of the
rubber dam in the approximal area, this may be overcome by
placing a hard wood wedge between the teeth; this will, over a
period of a few minutes, displace both the rubber dam and the
gingival tissues apically. The use of such a wedge will also reduce
the likelihood of injuring the soft tissues or of tearing the rubber
dam with rotary instruments.

Operative procedure. The position of the carious lesion should
be determined and access to the lesion created by use of a tung-
sten carbide bur, such as a No. 56 or 170, in a friction-grip
handpiece at the correct level perpendicular to the long axis of the
tooth. Once the carious lesion is reached, the caries may be
excavated by use of a slowly-rotating round steel bur. If access
between the tooth to be restored and the one adjacent to it is
poor, the cavity may be more suitably restored using amalgam
rather than glass ionomer cement. If this is the case, mechanical
retention following caries removal must be devised. The most
suitable sites for this are in the axio-gingival and axio-occlusal
line angles, where retention grooves may be placed using a
half-round steel bur. These grooves should be more definite at
the more distant part of the preparation in order to provide
retention against lateral displacement of the restoration (Fig.
6.3). Prior to placing the amalgam restoration, a calcium hydroxide hard-setting base should be placed in the deeper portions of

a   b

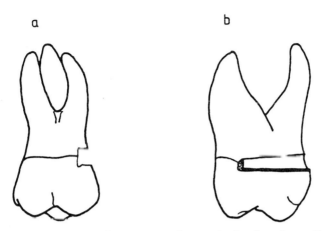

Fig 6.3   *Cavity preparation for restoration of approximal surface of upper first molar. (a) Buccal view of cavity showing retention grooves. (b) Mesial aspect showing slot preparation.*

the preparation, followed by three thin coats of copal ether varnish to reduce the early microleakage around the restoration.

Inserting the restoration. Matrix selection and placement is important if correct contour of the amalgam is to be achieved. The most suitable method is to use a strip of thin metal matrix band, which is wedged and supplemented by softened compound. This allows condensation with small condensers, such as a 1S, to be carried out through the initial access site prepared at the facial or lingual line angle of the tooth. Following condensation and removal of the matrix, the restoration should be checked to ensure that any excess amalgam is removed and that the correct contour has been produced. Amalgam restorations, particularly in this area, should be smoothed and finished at a subsequent visit in order to facilitate the patient's plaque control procedures. Where access to approximal lesions is less difficult, glass ionomer cement with its adhesive and cariostatic properties would be the preferred restorative material.

Secondary caries

Diagnosis

At one extreme, the diagnosis of secondary caries may be easy, e.g. when a new lesion is obviously associated with an existing

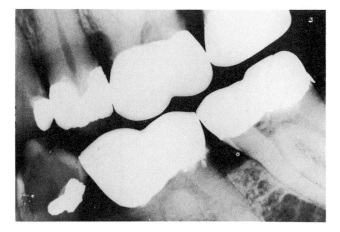

Fig 6.4   *Bitewing radiograph showing radiolucencies mesially* 6 *and distally* 6. *Neither of these proved to be due to dental caries.*

restoration. In the absence of such an obvious sign, discoloura- tion of tooth structure adjacent to a restoration may be associated with recurrent caries, but this is not an absolute diagnostic criterion. The diagnosis of recurrent caries requires a thorough clinical examination under good illumination with the teeth dry. Examination of root surfaces for recurrent caries, or lesions occurring *de novo*, is complicated by the fact that normal cemen- tum is slightly softer than sound dentine.

This may convey the impression of slight softening, even when the tissues are sound. Lesions of root caries generally progress relatively slowly, and re-examination of such doubtful areas at a later date will confirm whether there is in fact a progressive lesion. Radiographs are essential to aid diagnosis of carious lesions; intra-oral bitewing radiographs are more infor- mative than periapicals. Care must be taken in interpreting them since caries associated with metallic restorations may be difficult to see radiographically. Occasionally carious lesions in the gin- gival third of the tooth or on approximal root surfaces may be erroneously interpreted as 'cervical burnout' (Fig. 6.4).

Another indication of secondary caries is the marginal integ- rity of a restoration; loss of marginal integrity with a resin restoration certainly provides grounds for removal and assess- ment. However, the same criterion applied to amalgam restora- tions may result in the patient suffering a needless restorative procedure. 'Ditched' amalgam margins are an extremely common finding and the reasons for their appearance include creep (time-dependent deformation under load) or corrosion of the amalgam. Both of these phenomena lead to deflection of the margin of the restoration, subsequent fracture in this area, and hence 'ditching' or loss of marginal integrity. Despite this loss of marginal integrity, amalgam restorations have been shown to permit decreased microleakage with time. The reasons for this are related either to the deposition of products of corrosion in the tooth-restoration interface, or to the fact that marginal integrity is only lost in the cavo-surface area and thus does not affect the overall seal of the restoration. This presents a dilemma: whether or not to remove such an amalgam restoration on the grounds that there may be secondary caries present. This is where such factors as inspection with the teeth dry under a good light, and signs of marked discolouration adjacent to the amalgam, are of importance. If there is no evidence of secondary caries other than a 'ditched' margin of an amalgam restoration, it would seem prudent to leave the restoration and to re-assess at a later visit.

It is salutary to remember that the most common cause of ditched amalgam margins is not poor performance of the material, but rather the failure of the clinician to produce a 90° angle of amalgam in the marginal area. The angle most commonly created is more acute, which predisposes the amalgam to marginal fracture (Elderton 1984).

When such an amalgam restoration is replaced there is often little tendency to modify the preparation to produce a better marginal angle of amalgam, thus predisposing the restoration to recurrent loss of marginal integrity and repeated replacement. Thus, when any cavity preparation for amalgam is made, the

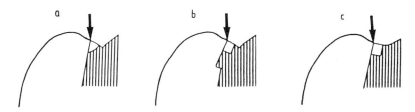

Fig 6.5   *(a) Incorrect cavity design leading to an acute angle of amalgam at the margin. This should be modified either by (b) further cavity preparation or by (c) less severe carving of the isthmus where the occlusion permits. Both of these modifications will produce an amalgam margin closer to 90°.*

isthmus of the preparation must be examined and, if necessary, the marginal area modified to create the correct cavosurface angle, as shown in Fig. 6.5.

FRACTURE OF TEETH

Elderly patients commonly suffer from fracture of the teeth without a history of trauma. These may range from chipping of the incisal edge of an anterior tooth, or loss of a single cusp of a posterior tooth, to complete loss of the clinical crown which is seen most commonly in the anterior region of the mouth. Incomplete fractures, involving both the root and crown of a tooth, may cause symptoms of pain or mobility of the teeth: alternatively, the signs and symptoms of a periodontal abscess or a sudden increase in pocket depth may be the first indication that such an event has taken place. Occasionally a patient may complain of intermittent pain, often severe, from a posterior tooth on chewing. On initial examination, even radiologically, the tooth appears both vital and intact, but further investigation discloses a crack in the dentine which is responsible for the symptoms.

If external trauma, such as a blow to the tooth, is excluded, the factors responsible may be:

1. Age changes in the dental tissues.
2. The effect of previous restorations.
3. Occlusal factors.

Age changes in dental tissues

Age changes in the dental tissues are discussed in Chapter 2. Although these changes may contribute towards the tendency of teeth in elderly patients to fracture spontaneously, in most instances clinical observation would suggest that their role is contributory rather than predominant.

The effects of previous restorations and the prevention of fractures

The concept that restorations are capable of 'reinforcing' teeth is implied in many dental textbooks. The most widely-known example of reinforcement is the use of a post inserted into the root canal of an endodontically treated tooth. The literature on this subject is equivocal. On the one hand there is some evidence from laboratory studies that teeth with posts fracture at slightly higher loads than similar teeth without posts. However, the theory has been suggested that under such circumstances the post simply helps to distribute the load throughout the root rather than providing reinforcement. Most research into the effects of cavity preparation indicates that operative procedures which remove dental hard tissues weaken teeth. In particular, it has been demonstrated that increasing the width of isthmus of a cavity preparation significantly reduces the resistance to fracture of that tooth.

Many of the anterior teeth which suffer complete fracture of the clinical crown are found to have Class V or Class III restorations below the level of the cement–enamel junction. The discussion on root caries has already highlighted the lack of dentine in areas apical to the anatomical crown of the tooth. If the bulk of dentine in these areas has been reduced further by cavity preparation, it is easy to understand how such teeth may fracture, particularly if the effects of increased mechanical stress related to an increase in clinical crown length are borne in mind.

Cuspal fracture of posterior teeth is not the exclusive province of the elderly. Nevertheless, there is a high incidence of the condition in this age group. Occasional fractures of this type are found in unrestored posterior teeth, but the vast majority can usually be attributed to faulty management of previous restorative procedures. Where cavity preparation has involved the creation of a wide and/or deep isthmus, the support for the remaining cusps must be considered. It is to be stressed that amalgam or any other restorative material, when used intracoronally, is incapable of supporting weakened enamel or dentine. Nevertheless, clinicians are reluctant to reduce unsupported cusps and overlay them with at least 2mm of amalgam. This reluctance to sacrifice 'sound' tooth structure is understandable, particularly when the aesthetics of the tooth may be compromised. However, failure to produce cuspal protection may predispose the tooth to later fracture, which will happen in an uncontrolled manner and may be catastrophic for the tooth and in particular for the patient.

Clinical observation suggests that the incidence of tooth fracture is increasing. This may simply be a reflection of the fact that people are retaining their teeth for longer periods. It is now felt, with justification, that teeth need not necessarily be lost as age increases. This change in the pattern of dental disease places more responsibility on the clinician to create restorations which do not predispose to failure of the teeth or supporting structures. With regard to operative treatment of carious lesions, concepts of what constitutes ideal cavity preparation require re-evaluation. Many of the changes in cavity design are covered by consideration of the treatment of a simple Class II carious lesion. A carious lesion in enamel does not require operative intervention unless there is evidence of dentinal spread. If an enamel lesion is discovered during routine examination, it should be treated in a preventive manner by dietary control, attention to plaque control and the use of topical fluorides. Many of these lesions never progress and, until evidence of dentinal spread is obtained at a later recall appointment, no cavity preparation should be carried out. When a carious lesion demands treatment, it must be borne in mind that if the restoration is to be of benefit to the patient it should not render the tooth more liable to fracture or periodontal disease. The concept of minimal cavity preparation is not new and is well documented in some of the more recent textbooks on Operative Dentistry. The basic features of such a cavity preparation are illustrated in Fig. 6.6. There is no requirement to make an isthmus unless there is caries present occlusally, or an existing amalgam restoration, or a deep fissure pattern which is at risk from carious attack. If an isthmus is to be prepared, it should be as narrow as possible, approximately 0.8–1.0mm wide and just into dentine; it should have rounded internal form and allow

a   b

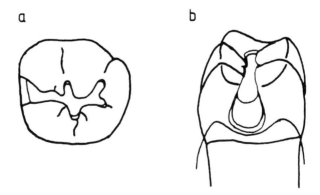

Fig 6.6   *Class II cavity preparation for amalgam. (a) Occlusal view showing minimal extension. (b) Mesial view illustrating rounded internal form with approximal box conforming to the shape of the contact area and gingival tissues.*

creation of a 90° amalgam margin angle. The approximal box should be rounded or teardrop-shaped in outline in order to conform to the shape of the interdental space, with minimal bucco-lingual and gingival extension – no more than is sufficient to allow access to the margins for finishing purposes. The internal form of such cavities will be rounded in order to reduce the stress concentration within both the tooth and the restorative material.

This current concept of cavity design recognises certain factors from the dental literature. The concept of 'extension for prevention' is no longer valid, for there is no evidence that production of a large restoration prevents secondary dental caries. The existence of self-cleansing areas is also not held to be valid; numerous studies have demonstrated that self-cleansing action is minimal and, where present, is confined to the occlusal one-third of the clinical crowns of the teeth. In addition, there is no indication for the extension of sound cavity margins into sub-gingival areas; no benefit is gained with regard to the prevention of recurrent dental caries, whilst sub-gingival restoration margins have been clearly correlated with increased levels of gingival inflammation (Renggli and Regolati 1972).

Where more extensive restorations are indicated, the rounded internal form of a minimal amalgam preparation will not provide adequate retention and resistance form. Under these circumstances, sharp internal line angles should be produced in the preparation.

Indications for the use of pins

Where cusps are missing, retention and resistance form is not easily achieved. The ease with which retentive amalgam restorations may be created by the use of pins tends to lead to their ill-considered use. When Markley first introduced cemented dentine pins, he suggested that they reinforced amalgam in the same way that concrete could be reinforced with steel rods. It is now known that pins actually weaken the amalgam. Cemented pins require insertion depths of at least 3mm and are time-consuming to use. The introduction of friction-lock and, in particular, self-threading pins has made the use of pins relatively straightforward. However, both these latter types of pin create stresses within the tooth structure and, remembering that dentine in the elderly has increased brittleness, they must be used with extreme caution and in minimal quantity. Strenuous attempts must be made to produce maximal retention and resistance form in cavity design, using such features as boxes, grooves and rails. If, having done all this, retention is still inadequate then auxiliary pin retention is indicated, with a maximum of one pin placed per missing cusp. The pin should be bent to provide opposing wall retention and also to lie completely within the restorative material. Where the teeth are particularly brittle or weakened, the use of pins should be avoided and, in the case of teeth treated endodontically, the root canals should be used to gain retention. Where pin retention is unavoidable in brittle teeth, cemented pins, which do not create installation stresses, should be used.

The use of pins for the restoration of anterior teeth is often recommended, particularly when cavities involve the incisal edge of the tooth. This practice has little to commend it: there is little dentine available for pin placement, particularly if the teeth have long clinical crowns, whilst the acid-etched enamel technique for use with composite resins has made such procedures generally obsolete. Pin-retained amalgam restorations may be very useful for elderly patients in providing a method of restoring broken down or fractured teeth to function. Well executed, they can sometimes provide an alternative to castings for posterior teeth. However, even with good cuspal coverage by amalgam, they do not provide the same degree of protection for the remaining tooth structure as a cast metal veneer. For the majority of restorations where pin retention is indicated, the self-threading pin is generally preferred, having the advantages of ease of placement together with good retentive properties. Selection of the appropriate size of self-threading pin is important. Most elderly patients show increased length of clinical crowns. The most likely area in which to place pins therefore lies at or apical to the cement–enamel junction, where there is only a small bulk of dentine between the periodontal ligament and the root canal of the tooth. The selection of appropriate sites is important, and these have been represented in Fig. 6.7. The standard size of most self-threading pins is of the order of 0.7mm. Most manufacturers offer a number of pin diameters, and it would thus seem prudent to use pins of smaller diameters to avoid the risk of either periodontal or pulpal perforation. A pin size of approximately 0.6mm is generally suitable for all molar and most premolar teeth.

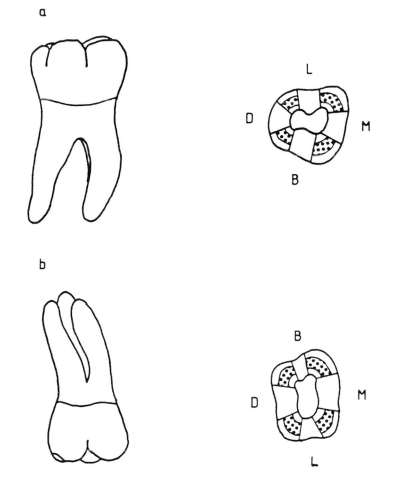

Fig 6.7   *Cross-sections taken at the level of the cement–enamel junction. (a) Lower first molar. (b) Upper first molar. Shaded areas indicate favourable locations for pins in molar teeth.*

Occlusal considerations

The forces produced by the masticatory muscles often appear to be sufficient to fracture even the strongest available restorative material. It is a clinical observation that many restorations placed without due consideration of contacts occurring both on closing and in excursive movements of the mandible suffer fracture. In addition, tooth fracture may be associated with teeth which constitute interferences to mandibular movement. The subject of occlusion is not one that can be dealt with in depth in a text of this type. However, some fundamental principles may be used to guide the clinician in occlusal management for operative procedures. Occlusal requirements for natural teeth are different from those for complete dentures. It is felt that the natural dentition should demonstrate multiple, even contacts between the posterior teeth when the patient closes. It is considered desirable that, when the mandible moves, the teeth on the side away from which the mandible is moving should be out of contact. In a protrusive movement, it is also considered desirable that the posterior teeth should separate. The presence of non-working contacts may interfere with smooth mandibular movement. Such contacts place heavy loads obliquely on the teeth, which may result in the fracture of cusps or restorations. The simple expedient of examining posterior teeth prior to and after restoration, to ensure that non-working side interferences are absent, may provide considerable rewards in preventing tooth or restoration fracture.

Another common problem is that of an amalgam restoration which fractures repeatedly. One solution often suggested is to deepen the isthmus in order to increase the bulk of restorative material. The result may be a restoration which remains intact, but only at the cost of sacrificing tooth substance and so increasing subsequent vulnerability to fracture. In the majority of such cases, if the restoration and the opposing tooth are examined, it will be found that the restoration exhibits a deep fossa whilst the opposing cusp is over-erupted relative to the occlusal plane of the arch.

Such over-erupted cusps are potent causes of non-working-side interferences on mandibular movement and, by the simple expedient of reducing them, an increased bulk of material can be incorporated into the new restoration. Therefore, the benefits of modifying the opposing tooth will be an increased bulk of restorative material without further weakening of the tooth, together with a reduction in the potential for fracture of the tooth or restoration resulting from occlusal interferences.

TOOTH WEAR

Tooth wear is a common finding in the elderly. In this chapter, only the treatment of wear will be dealt with. Different types of tooth wear and their causes are dealt with in Chapter 2.

Abrasion

It is important that the condition, once diagnosed, is not allowed to persist for too long, otherwise structural weakening of the teeth may take place, predisposing them to fracture. Attempts should be made to modify the tooth-brushing technique used by the patient, in order to prevent a horizontal scrubbing method being used over the gingival portion of the teeth. This will sometimes be difficult to achieve where such habits have been established over many years. Existing abrasion lesions of significant depth should be restored with glass ionomer cement, which will adhere to the dentine of the root surface. It is preferable that, if abrasion continues, it is the restorative material that is worn away rather than further sound tooth structure.

Erosion

The control of the aetiological factors is of considerable importance. This may involve modification of the diet for extrinsic causes or medical management where an intrinsic factor has been found. Strict attention to oral hygiene procedures, in combination with a desensitising toothpaste, will reduce pain from thermal, tactile and osmotic stimuli. Eroded areas on the facial or lingual surfaces of teeth may be restored with glass ionomer cement or, if the lesions have margins in enamel, with acid-etch-retained composite resin restorations. Application of desensitising agents may prove beneficial. Many of these may be damaging to the pulp; one effective and non-toxic agent, however, is a fluoride-containing varnish which is applied to the dried surface of the erosion lesion. The use of acidified fluoride solutions is inadvisable, as their low pH may cause further loss of dentine.

The management of sensitivity may be enhanced by instructing the patient to rub a small quantity of desensitising toothpaste into the erosion lesion with a finger and allow the paste to remain in contact with the tooth for five to ten minutes prior to brushing. Those patients who suffer from acid regurgitation, particularly at night, or who have to take acid regularly for achlorhydria, may require protection for their teeth. This may be achieved by the construction of vacuum-formed soft vinyl bite guards to cover the teeth. These may be coated internally with an alkali such as magnesium hydroxide and worn either at night or prior to taking acid. The management of erosion of the occlusal surfaces of the teeth presents greater problems, and will be discussed in the section dealing with extensive wear.

Attrition

Some wear of the functioning surfaces of the teeth would be expected in elderly patients. Wear that is slight in proportion to the patient's age, and not causing symptoms, requires no active treatment. However, the patient should be examined at recall appointments to determine whether any significant change has taken place. It is helpful in this respect to make impressions for study casts, which can be retained. This will allow comparisons to be made at subsequent visits.

The role of dental materials in tooth wear

Reference has already been made to simple occlusal management for restorative dentistry. However, it is also important that the restorations themselves do not induce further wear. Macrofilled composite resins are considered unsuitable for the restoration of the occlusal surfaces of posterior teeth, since they abrade rapidly. It is not generally known that they will also abrade opposing enamel and dentine. Large Class III and Class IV anterior composite restorations will do the same to lower incisor teeth and, on this basis, the microfilled composites which are less abrasive are perhaps more suitable.

The occlusal surfaces of posterior teeth should, wherever possible, be restored with metal. Porcelain is potentially highly abrasive to opposing teeth, whether these are unrestored or have metal restorations. Amalgam or gold produce relatively little wear either of each other or of opposing tooth structure. In addition, laboratory waxing techniques for cast gold restorations permit greater accuracy of occlusal form than can generally be achieved using porcelain.

Management of extensive wear

Marked wear of the teeth, whether by attrition alone or in

combination with erosion of the occlusal surfaces, may present both functional and aesthetic problems. Restoring the heavily worn dentition in the elderly is a difficult task. The choice of treatment will depend largely on the patient's health, both physical and dental, and his attitude and wishes. It is not correct to think that extensive cast restorations are contra-indicated for elderly patients. For some, this may be one of the finest services the dentist can provide. Techniques for comprehensive occlusal rehabilitation are to be found in most text books dealing with the subject of occlusion.

Patients with slight to moderate wear can usually be managed in a relatively conservative way. This may involve some restorations, either intra- or extra-coronally, together with the provision of an occlusal splint to be worn at night to protect the teeth when clenching and grinding habits are involved in the process of wear. Such occlusal appliances should provide stable occlusal contacts for all the opposing teeth, in order that no irreversible changes in the occlusion are caused by some teeth being out of contact with the appliance and consequently at risk of over-eruption. The area in which the dentist can make the maximal contribution in terms of management of tooth wear is in preventing the advanced occlusal wear which necessitates extensive treatment. It is important that all adult patients are routinely assessed for the degree of tooth wear relative to their age. If signs of excessive wear are found, the patient requires therapy, either by occlusal appliances, by occlusal adjustment, or possibly by subsequent tooth restoration.

ENDODONTICS

The pulp of a tooth in an elderly patient is only a little younger than the patient. Age changes occur in both patients and their dental tissues and the dental pulp is no exception. Age changes of the pulp are discussed in Chapter 2. Pulp vitality will be affected by a decrease in the size and complexity of the vascular pattern and a decrease in cellularity. The vascular changes in particular affect the peripheral odontoblastic capillary plexus, which implies a decrease in odontoblastic activity. Thus the ability of the pulp to respond to insults is reduced.

The effects of dental caries, tooth wear and restorative procedures on the dental pulp are cumulative. Thus, the pulps of elderly patients may be severely compromised. Where restorative procedures are to be carried out emphasis should be placed on an atraumatic technique, with good control of the operating field to minimise bacterial contamination of the prepared tooth, adequate pulp protection, and the use of restorative materials causing minimal pulpal injury. It is not surprising that loss of pulp vitality is common in elderly patients. In such cases, access to the root canal system to carry out definitive endodontics may be difficult, since deposition of secondary dentine throughout life may have reduced the size of (or obliterated) the pulp chamber. In premolar and molar teeth, secondary dentine formation takes place preferentially on the floor and roof of the pulp chamber. In cases where the pulp chamber has been obliterated, the access cavity for endodontics may need to be prepared deeply enough to gain access directly into the root canals. This should be done with caution to minimise the risk of perforation. Deposition of secondary dentine may have narrowed or virtually obliterated root canals, whilst pulpal calcification may occasionally impede instrumentation. Despite these problems, endodontics can be successfully carried out for elderly patients.

Endodontic treatment may allow preservation of important teeth; the retention of anterior teeth may avoid the need for a prosthetic replacement to be constructed; successful endodontic treatment of a distal molar abutment may save the patient from the difficulties of a distal extension removable partial denture. Finally the retention of a few healthy roots may provide the foundation for an over-denture (see Chapter 7). Whenever endodontics is undertaken, the final restoration must be considered. Endodontic procedures involve loss of a considerable amount of coronal and radicular tooth structure, with consequent weakening of the teeth. In premolars and molar teeth, restorations placed intra-coronally will produce wedging forces between the buccal and lingual cusps. Posterior teeth restored in this manner have an increased tendency to split. All such endodontically treated posterior teeth should receive restorations that provide cuspal coverage; these restorations should be castings.

INDICATIONS FOR CAST RESTORATIONS AND TOOTH REPLACEMENT

Elderly patients, like any others, may benefit from strategic use of cast or veneer restorations. In the anterior region, the indications are either for aesthetic purposes (although composite resins have reduced the need for them), or for functional requirements in some cases of fractured, non-vital, or extremely worn teeth. Posteriorly, the aesthetic requirements are reduced, but cast restorations are indicated for cases where occlusal form is to be restored or for protection of remaining tooth structure.

There is obviously no indication for cast restorations as a method of preventing caries, and virtually none for their use in patients suffering from periodontal disease. Castings are not a treatment for any type of dental disease; they simply restore anatomical form and may protect the remaining tooth structure. The margins of cast restorations should, wherever possible, lie clear of the gingival tissues. If margins are placed close to marginal tissues, particular care must be taken to produce correct or somewhat flattened axial contours to allow the patient good access for plaque control. In addition, if periodontal health is not to be compromised, preparations and castings should take into account features such as molar furcations and root grooves.

Many of these considerations for cast restorations will apply to fixed tooth replacement. Each patient must be assessed to determine whether tooth replacement is necessary and, if it is, whether a fixed or removable appliance is indicated. Not all teeth which are lost require replacement. For example, in an elderly patient, loss of one or two posterior teeth may not necessitate the construction of a prosthesis if there are sufficient posterior teeth to allow function and occlusal stability to be maintained. However, the condition of the remaining dentition should be assessed. If further tooth loss is anticipated, it may be preferable to construct a partial denture so that the patient may become accustomed to wearing a prosthesis before a distal extension partial denture is required. Alternatively, it may be judged that such a prosthesis is unlikely to be necessary. The replacement of teeth is contra-indicated where no functional or aesthetic need exists. Consequently, in this area in particular, each elderly patient should be assessed in both the short and long term to determine present and future needs.

THE DIAGNOSIS OF CAUSES OF DENTAL PAIN

One aspect of the restorative needs of elderly patients that deserves particular consideration is the diagnosis of pain. Not all the causes of dental pain can be described here. However, it is intended to discuss those areas of diagnosis which are more pertinent to the elderly.

History

When an elderly patient complains of pain, as with all other patients, a history must be taken. If the patient is fit and alert, then this may not present too great a problem, but such may not always be the case. It is well known that a satisfactory diagnosis of the cause of dental pain is dependent on an adequate history. Therefore, questions should be clear and concise. In addition, it is important that the patient is given time to answer and, if there is difficulty in following the questions, they must be repeated or rephrased – but always in a kindly manner. For those patients who have difficulty in communicating the nature of the problem, it may be possible to enlist the help of those who help to look after them, either at home, in the Residential Home, or in hospital. Such relatives or nurses may be able to provide a history of the timing and duration of the pain, what foods are deliberately avoided, and whether the patient's sleep is disturbed.

Examination

The history, once obtained, should be followed by a thorough examination of the mouth, including the soft tissues, rather than being localised to the area where pain is perceived. This should be done in order to exclude the presence of disease elsewhere in the mouth and also to reduce the possibility that the examination will miss features that may be of importance to the diagnosis. Young, fit and healthy adults may often find it difficult to locate the site of their own dental pain: for the elderly patient, who is physically compromised and in some instances not mentally alert, these difficulties may be increased. The examination should take into account that a denture may be the cause of pain. It should therefore include an assessment of the dentures themselves and of the tissues which support them. The temporomandibular joints and their associated musculature should also be examined. In addition, pain from a vascular cause, the sinuses, malignancies, or atypical facial pain with no organic cause may also occur in patients of this age-group.

Pain of dental origin

When diagnosing dental pain in older patients, particularly those with natural teeth remaining, the examination may take longer and a conclusion may be less easily reached.

The dental pulp. Causes of dental pain may arise within the pulp or the periodontal ligament. The pulp in the elderly patient, as already discussed, is inevitably compromised. The effects of age changes, tooth wear, and previous restorative treatment will all have contributed to decrease the defence capacity of any remaining pulpal tissue. The result of this may be a tooth in which the pulp dies, giving rise to symptoms as it does so or, commonly, dying without symptoms and giving rise to pain at some later time.

Anaesthesia. Many elderly patients who require local anaesthesia for operative procedures are medically compromised. Individuals suffering from hypertension or ischaemic heart disease are often considered at risk from local anaesthetic agents containing adrenaline. This problem was reviewed by Cawson et al. (1983), who found little support for this view. However, the importance of effective anaesthesia is apparent, not only for patient comfort, but to minimise the cardiovascular effects of stress. Local anaesthesia should be provided for the elderly patient as necessary, although it is observed clinically that their teeth are often relatively insensitive during restorative procedures. Anaesthesia for a single tooth may be provided using an intraligamentary technique. This may be useful in aiding diagnosis of dental pain, or when regional anaesthesia is considered undesirable. Neither intravenous sedation nor general anaesthesia should be undertaken without recourse to specialists in these fields.

Cracked teeth. Tooth wear has already been discussed: this may give rise to pain from the teeth and, under some circumstances, from the temporomandibular joints and associated musculature. Cracks in teeth have also been mentioned earlier. These may present difficulties in diagnosis. Cracks present symptoms which are related to their extent and to the state of the pulp. Typically, a patient with a cracked tooth complains of pain from a posterior tooth that is increased momentarily when the pressure of chewing is relieved. Such symptoms imply a crack involving enamel and dentine only. If the pain also occurs with hot and cold substances, it usually indicates extension of the crack to involve the pulp. In the long term, such cracks may produce irreversible pulpal damage, with the appearance of symptoms of pain and swelling.

Inspection alone will not always reveal cracks. A useful diagnostic test is to place a small soft rubber polishing wheel between the suspected tooth and the antagonist and ask the patient to squeeze the teeth together firmly. Pain on release of the pressure is indicative of a cracked tooth. The diagnosis may be confirmed by removing the restoration under rubber dam and flowing disclosing solution into the cavity. This is washed away after one or two minutes, and the tooth is dried. Careful inspection may reveal the presence of a crack. Transillumination may also be used to reveal cracks in teeth, but this method is less reliable. In cases where there are no symptoms of irreversible pulpal damage, or where the diagnosis still remains in doubt, confirmation may be obtained by cementing a stainless steel orthodontic band or a trimmed and smoothed copper band around the tooth and placing a provisional restoration intra-coronally. Relief of the symptoms over a period of one or two weeks will confirm the diagnosis of a cracked tooth.

It is likely that many elderly patients will demonstrate the results of previous periodontal disease. The exposure of the roots of the teeth implies that root caries, particularly with direct pulpal involvement, may be a cause of pain. Careful examination is necessary to discover such lesions, particularly when they are situated on the approximal surfaces of teeth or in the furcation areas of molars.

Periodontal disease. The presence of periodontal disease may increase the possibility of pain due to a periodontal abscess. Whilst the effect of periodontal disease on the dental pulp is unproven, there is histological evidence that it may contribute to pulp ageing, so that periodontal disease with exposure of lateral or accessory root canals may make some contribution to pulp death.

Elderly patients may complain of pain from mobile teeth. It should be determined whether pain is due to inflammation apically or laterally within the periodontal ligament, or to lack of periodontal support. The latter is not usually a cause of pain unless the tooth is so mobile that it moves markedly and is thus tender on chewing. Where pulpal or periodontal inflammation is unlikely to be the cause of pain, examination of the lateral and protrusive movements may suggest that the mobility is being aggravated by an occlusal interference.

Special tests

These should be used to confirm or extend findings from the clinical examination. Pulp vitality may be assessed by several methods, none of which is completely reliable.

Pulp testers

These are said to be effective in the elderly patient, as there should be no change in conduction through elderly dentine. However, all the teeth in the suspected area should be tested to provide an indication of the general level of response. The pulp tester should be placed on sound, dry tooth structure. It should also be remembered that these instruments may interfere with the correct functioning of certain cardiac pacemakers.

Thermal tests

Tests with hot and cold substances, e.g. hot gutta percha and ice sticks, may be of value, but slower responses should be anticipated due to the increased thickness of dentine present in an older person's teeth.

Test cavities

In situations where difficulty is found in obtaining a response with electrical or thermal stimulation, the preparation of a small test cavity in sound tooth structure may be a helpful diagnostic aid. However, the increased bulk of dentine present may require a moderately deep cavity before a vital tooth will give a response.

Radiographs

Bitewing radiographs should be used to help diagnose approximal carious lesions. For examination of the periapical areas of the teeth, long cone radiographs should be taken to provide a less distorted image than will be produced by conventional bisecting angle views. The periodontal ligament space should be examined for signs of increased width that may indicate the effects of pulpal disease. However, it should be remembered that teeth which are mobile simply because of an increased crown:root ratio will show such widening of the periodontal ligament space as an adaptive feature.

This summarises some of the causes of dental pain which may be found in the elderly. However, it is emphasised that, even in this age group, dental caries will be a very common cause of pain. The importance of a good history, coupled with a careful examination, cannot be overstated.

COMPROMISE IN TREATMENT OF THE ELDERLY

This chapter has sought to deal with restorative procedures for the elderly patient. It is apparent that in most respects these are no different from restorative dentistry for any adult patient. Any differences are due to the altered disease patterns seen in this age-group. However, this chapter has necessarily assumed that the elderly patient is a relatively fit individual, who has good access to dental care, and this is indeed true of the majority of these patients. Nevertheless, there are many elderly patients whose age and infirmity make access to a dentist difficult, if not impossible, and whose tolerance of restorative procedures will be very low. These factors, either singly or in combination, demand some compromise in treatment.

'Compromise' in dentistry suggests a failure to carry out satisfactory work. This is only true if the dentist makes a compromise to suit himself; if, however, a compromise is decided upon after a complete diagnosis has been made, this cannot be regarded as a failure to treat satisfactorily. Indeed, it may represent a judgement of the patient's needs and how best to fulfil them. There will be patients for whom caries removal using an excavator followed by an intermediate zinc oxide–eugenol restoration will represent the appropriate treatment. In the same way, an extraction may be preferable to endodontic therapy.

In the treatment of the elderly, the need for compromise may arise from the patient's level of health, his wishes, his tolerance of dental procedures, and whether he has access to the dentist's practice, or whether he has to be treated at home or in hospital. The only area which should not give rise to compromise is that of the attitude of the dentist to the elderly; good quality restorative care is certainly possible for the majority of elderly patients, and the responsibility for this rests with the dentist.

REFERENCES

Axelsson P., Lindhe J. (1981). Effect of controlled oral hygiene procedures on caries and periodontal disease in adults. *J. Clin. Periodontol.*; **8**: 239–48.

Cawson R. A., Curson I., Whittington D. R. (1983). The hazards of dental local anaesthetics. *Br. Dent. J.*; **154**: 253–8.

Elderton R. J. (1984). Cavo-surface angles, amalgam margin angles and occlusal cavity preparations. *Br. Dent. J.*; **156**: 319–24.

King J. M., Hardie J. M., Duckworth R. (1985). Dental caries and periodontal health following a professionally administered plaque control programme in adolescents. *Br. Dent. J.*; **158**: 52–4.

Renggli H. H., Regolati B. (1972). Gingival inflammation and plaque accumulation by well-adapted supra-gingival and subgingival proximal restorations. *Helv. Odont. Acta*; **16**: 99–101.

Chapter 7

The Management of Missing Teeth
H. THOMSON

INTRODUCTION

Loss of teeth at any age can either be demoralising or a welcome relief from pain. In the elderly of today, who were young when extractions were the treatment for toothache, it may still be acceptable as inevitable. However, dental health education in the past 30 years has reached most generations and today's elderly justifiably protest, for the most part, against any but the most necessary loss of teeth. These elderly people are not only increasing in number – with some living to a great age – but are finding that their income is not always related to the cost of living and certainly not to the cost of dentistry. They also have disabilities and illness, with consequent difficulty in getting to the dentist, and in many cases they are confined to homes or institutions. Dental care for these people, some of whom urgently require it, can therefore be difficult to provide. Dentists may also find that their appointment books are full enough, without having to provide for this neglected population. Some of these patients give up the struggle of trying to find a dentist who will care for them, and accept limited mouth function as part of becoming old. Others are tireless in their quest for improved eating efficiency and appearance and, as these two factors are important to survival and morale, their needs must be served.

The concept of caring, when applied to dental care for the elderly, implies enquiring about their dental needs, advising on preventive measures and providing treatment where necessary. This chapter will therefore deal with reasons for difficulties in replacing teeth for the elderly, with attitudes and planning, with the problems and needs arising from the retention of a few teeth, and with the possibilities of providing treatment in home or institution. Some details will be given on partial denture design, overdentures, the transition to complete dentures, the elderly edentulous patient with unsatisfactory dentures, improvement procedures, the problems of providing new dentures, and the present status of implants.

Tissue changes

What is the difference between treating elderly and younger patients with few or no teeth? The answer lies partly in cellular changes that take place in the ageing organism, as a consequence of which the process of cell renewal dwindles to a halt. Loss of hair is a common example. Cells of ageing mucosal surfaces are not readily replaced, and tissues are less robust as a consequence; this is especially so in females, who are more subject to atrophic changes. Reception of stimuli and transmission of impulses become reduced and reactions are slower as a result; the five senses deteriorate, and the anticipated efficiency of new dentures may be affected by the loss of taste and touch. Muscle activities become impaired and this may affect the ability to control removable dentures. On the other hand, hyperactivity of the masticatory muscles may cause clenching of the teeth – both natural and artificial – and grinding movements of the mandibular teeth may follow, resulting in forces being transmitted to the ridges of residual bone with consequent resorption of the denture-bearing surfaces. This may also be destructive to any remaining teeth and their supporting tissues, and to the muscles themselves. The teeth, when present, become progressively more mineralised and are therefore more brittle and liable to fracture. This is especially likely where clenching and grinding habits have been established. Thus the tissues involved in supporting both partial and complete dentures are liable to change in the elderly patient. Both cause and effect can be difficult to control, however willing the patient may be to cooperate. Secretion of saliva diminishes and this can cause discomfort in the wearing of dentures. Facial skin loses its elasticity and wrinkles appear. Appeals to plump out denture surfaces and to advance the teeth can only provide a partial improvement since wrinkles are due to changes in the tissue and not to loss of teeth. When denture teeth are moved forwards, the stability of the denture can be impaired, but the patient seldom believes this protest by the dentist and insists on changes for reasons of appearance. Thus prosthodontics may become compromisodontics.

Home care by the patient

Lack of general health care, under-nourishment and neglect of hygiene will affect the attitude and cooperation of the elderly patient. Maintenance of appliances and of abutment teeth is not a task that can be undertaken easily in patients approaching the age of 80. Finger facility has deteriorated and bathroom design is not always suited to doing what the dentist prescribes; shopping for hygiene aids can be difficult to organise; and discouragement often follows. A visit by the dentist to the patient's home can be helpful for the purpose of getting the patient organised and making suggestions for home care with the facilities available. If dentures are being planned, the consultation may be carried out at that time and preliminary impressions made.

Care for those confined to home or institutions

This constitutes an aspect of dentistry which has not been comprehensively organised and it is left to individual practitioners and community services to provide domiciliary dental services. Some dental schools are arranging for students or graduates to treat patients in their homes but a greater awareness of this need is required. 'Visiting dentistry', 'domiciliary care' or 'gerodontics' are subjects being introduced as undergraduate courses in some dental schools, and students are being taken into homes and institutions in order to realise the difficulties and to plan facilities (see Chapter 5). Portable equipment is being designed by enthusiasts, but manufacturers are understandably reluctant to start production for a small demand. Boxes and specialised instrument cases are available and experience by the individual practitioner will determine what to put in them. Portable dental motors are available but are not easy to use on patients away from the dental surgery. They are, of course, invaluable for denture work where trial bases have to be trimmed, over-extensions relieved, and occlusions adjusted. Discussions with illustrations will be included in the sections on procedures.

The elderly as patients

Old people can be difficult to treat. They can be psychologically disturbed as well as physically disabled, and they may be undergoing treatment for systemic conditions. The dentist can thus serve as a sounding board for their health and emotional problems, their worries, irrational fears and criticisms, especially if the dentist is compassionate and a good listener. These, of course, are two of the qualities required when treating the elderly. Consequently, the dentist must control the relationship so that the patient feels at ease but under treatment. Impatience should never be expressed, nor should the attitude reveal that short-term treatment will suffice because the patient is not going to live much longer. The advice to 'think patiently' has been given in Chapter 1 and this is precisely what is required when planning treatment for these patients. There are, on the other hand, patients in their seventies who have good health and many teeth but may well have complex dental problems. They may naturally wish to maintain and restore a youthful appearance, and may demand dentistry more suited to the middle aged. Care should be taken when planning treatment not to be too optimistic about brittle dentine or shrunken pulps when assessing bridge or denture abutments (see Chapter 6). Equally, periodontal tissues should be rendered secure for masticatory as well as abutment function. This may involve decisions on the wisdom of saving doubtful teeth and it may be necessary to employ specialist skill and experience before deciding the final plan. Associated with the dental plan are the factors of time, cost and prospects for compromise, even to the extent of leaving well alone. Old people, however, are sensitive to attitudes and have a life's experience of advising and being advised. They can tell when they are receiving less than they deserve, or think they deserve. Tact, compassion and skill are qualities required when advising as well as treating the elderly.

Retention of a few remaining teeth

The elderly are no different from the middle-aged in pleading for the retention of a few remaining teeth, especially in the mandibular arch. This arises from the much-publicised fear of an unstable mandibular denture. And dentists themselves share their apprehension. Whether for use as abutments for partial denture retainers, root supports for overlay dentures, or crowns for precision attachments, these remaining teeth can be precious. Dentists who are skilled and experienced in making dentures are often tempted to persuade elderly patients to accept the inevitable loss of suspect teeth at an age when their orofacial muscles are better able to adapt to and use the complete denture. In terms of persuasion the plea is often made that 'the younger you are the better you will be able to cope'. The dilemma is not easily solved: success and failure have been reported following decisions either way.

Retention of a few remaining teeth has to be viewed in terms of what is expected of them and what their response will be to load, torque, food stagnation and plaque. Also important, in their prognosis, is the shape and condition of the gingival and periodontal tissues and of the hard tissues themselves. Root-filled teeth are more brittle than those that are still vital, and their apical conditions should be viewed with critical concern. Finally, root surfaces are extremely susceptible to caries. In spite of all warning signs the patient will still want to save a lone tooth or both mandibular canines if for no other reason than for the feel of natural teeth which transmit the stimuli of vitality. Such pleas should be heeded.

Paying for services

Not least in the list of discouraging factors when treating the elderly is that of payment for services. Many a consultation with such a patient ends with the patient saying, 'You realise, of course, that I am on a pension'; and, whether the State, an insurance source, or the patient is paying, the factor of cost plays a part. Simple procedures and a kindly attitude are working maxims but not always practicable, and what is best is not always feasible. What follows are outlines of procedures which may prove successful with cost often being the factor determining choice.

PARTIAL DENTURES

Requirements

Many partial dentures reside in the handbag or pocket, to be worn for appearance (if front teeth are involved), and are often consigned to a box in a bottom drawer. They show signs of adjustments and are often a regretted extravagance. Design of these appliances for the elderly should not differ from the orthodox except that wrought wire retainers are often preferred to those of cast metal. Gold is also preferred to stainless steel for the reason of flexibility. This quality, however, can be improved in stainless steel by increasing the length of the retainer by a double coil where the wire emerges from the processed acrylic resin. This has been suggested by Dyer and is illustrated in

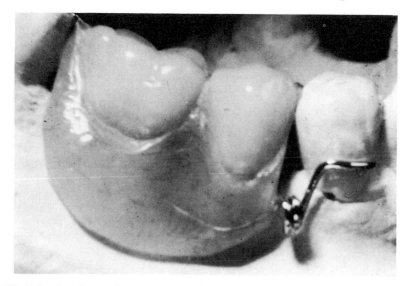

Fig 7.1   *Stainless steel wire retainer with double coil for increased flexibility. (Dyer, personal communication.)*

Fig. 7.1. However, no retainer should be designed without analysis on a surveyor table in order to assess the most favourable path of insertion and site of undercut. Acrylic resin bases are commonly preferred to cast metal for reasons of ease in achieving extension into areas of displaceable mucosa and fixation of wrought retainers. Where possible, coverage of the gingival tissue adjacent to the teeth should be avoided because these quickly become stagnation areas and the gingival margins become subject to inflammation by intermittent pressure.

There are three further requirements:

1. Replacement of teeth should be in the positions of their natural predecessors.

2. The intercuspal position of the mandible should be at the existing intercuspal position, unless there is an obvious and harmful displacement of the mandible on closure to intercuspal position by the existing natural teeth. Any interference (often caused by migrated teeth) giving rise to this displacement should be corrected by occlusal adjustment before making the final impressions.

3. The patient should be unaware of any uncomfortable occlusal change at intercuspal position; occlusal adjustment should therefore be made only after careful occlusal analysis.

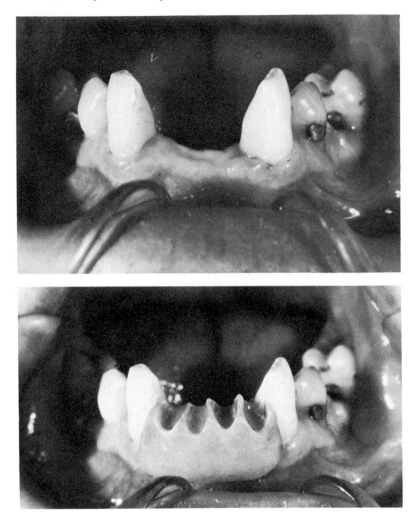

Fig 7.2   *The two part denture: (a) Removable denture required (b) Acrylic resin*

Muscle adaptability can be difficult for the older patient but a partial denture made to incorporate an existing occlusal disability may be less well tolerated and is often discarded for this reason.

Sometimes no denture at all, or the replacement of only front teeth, can be preferable to a costly venture into a reconstructed dentition. Decisions can be difficult and optimism should be tempered with reality.

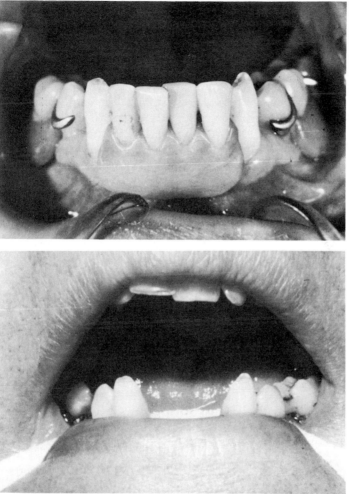

insert as part 1 (c) Denture inserted (d) Towelling the abutment teeth.

Developments

Five developments in partial denture design may help to solve special problems that will be described briefly.

1. The two-part denture (Fig. 7.2)

This can provide comfort and stability in a situation where tilted teeth adjacent to the saddle make denture insertion difficult and the prevention of stagnation almost impossible. The teeth are set in their desired positions with a space of at least 5mm between their necks and the supporting mucosa. This part of the denture, including retainers and other saddle areas, is then processed and completed. The gingival support segment is then waxed so that its path of insertion is from the labial (or buccal) aspect and, when processed, it is inserted first. The remainder of the denture is inserted from the occlusal direction, and locks the labial insert in place while permitting slight movement between the two parts and reducing stagnation. Care has to be taken to avoid losing the insert and it is advisable to make a spare at the outset. If the master cast is retained, further inserts can be made, but this will entail returning the denture to the laboratory. Alternatively, the inserts can be waxed in the mouth and subsequently processed.

2. The locking denture

The locking principle can be introduced to join the two parts on a hinge running between the abutment teeth. A metal tube is processed into the main part of the denture and a sliding bolt into the rotating insert. This is described by L'Estrange and Pullen–Warner (1969) and has proved successful for elderly patients especially when it has been provided in advance of age 70. The patient can then learn to manage the bolt while the fingers are still mobile. Needless to say, it is costly to produce.

3. The rotational path of insertion denture

This consists of a cast metal framework with a preliminary position of insertion at an axis of rotation determined by the surveyor and usually in the anterior segment. The casting is then rotated to place, when a minor connector engages the undercut below the survey line and provides retention. Conventional retainers can be used distally. This is described in detail by Jacobson and Krol (1982). Advantages include the utilisation of approximal undercuts, a reduction in the number and display of retainers and less exposed surface for plaque deposit in stagnation areas. An example is shown in Fig. 7.3.

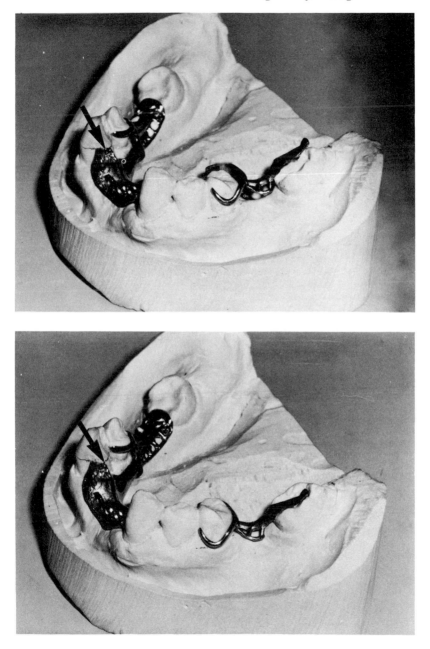

Fig 7.3   *The rotational path of insertion; (a) Casting rotating on 13 (b) Casting rotated into place.*

4. The Every denture

This is a denture of simple design, with no retainers but conforming strictly to certain principles. Designed by Every, it is described by Craddock (1956) and derives its retention from secure contact between the denture teeth and abutment teeth at their greatest convexities. A surveyor analysis of the cast is again important for design. Short lengths of steel wire inserted into the denture teeth adjacent to the abutment teeth at their greatest convexities are recommended in order to maintain the security of the contact. Two further features of design are emphasised: accuracy of adaptation of the denture base to the mucosa and no coverage of the gingival margins of the teeth. This denture is best utilised for the maxillary arch where the palate can be indented to provide a seal. This procedure is not recommended for the mucosa of the buccal sulcus, where the vertical movement of the denture during function would result in bruising. For the mandibular arch, retention is dependent on secure contact between

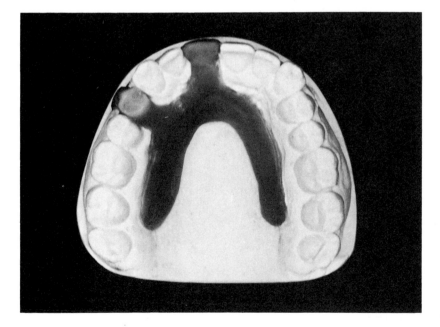

Fig 7.4   *The 'fork' partial denture.*

pontic and abutment teeth. As always, occlusal contacts between opposing teeth by cusp–fossa relations will provide efficiency in function and stability when the teeth are closed for swallowing.

5. The spoon denture

Finally there is the spoon, which needs no introduction and can provide a stable base for one or two missing teeth. A premolar may be added on one or both sides and the spoon may become a fork (Fig. 7.4) if the mid-part of the palate is too sensitive. The design should provide for the best possible seal. The labial gum should be extended above the neck of the incisor tooth and as far laterally as will be compatible with insertion and comfort.

Hygiene

This quality can deteriorate in the elderly where there is loneliness, confinement to home or institution, and no grandchildren to come visiting. But when the latter do come they can be the first to point out deficiencies and stains in the dentition. The use of dental tape and woodsticks may be easy for the more nimble-fingered under-seventies but may be difficult for the elderly, especially if they are being introduced to these measures for the first time. The effects of poor interdental hygiene can be explained to patients, and somehow they have got to keep these spaces clean. This can be done by instructing the patient to use a length of cotton bandage in a manner best described as 'towelling the teeth'. There is no better home-care method of cleaning cementum or exposed dentine and the method can be extended to other surfaces and spaces. Fluoridated toothpaste will help to prevent root caries and this should be an added incentive to hygiene. As to denture hygiene, a solution can be made from 4 teaspoonfuls of a powdered water-softener to one pint of water and from this solution two teaspoonfuls are added to a weak solution (1 teaspoonful to ¼ pint of water) of a 2% sodium hypochlorite w/v solution (Milton). Dentures (excluding those with base metal retainers or connectors) steeped in this solution overnight will remain clean and deposits of calculus will be reduced. An ultrasonic cleaning bath from time to time will help in getting rid of heavier deposits if patients can bring or send their dentures.

Occlusal habits

Contact between opposing teeth in the empty mouth disturbs dentures and their supporting teeth, and elderly patients do not respond easily to strictures on keeping their teeth apart. 'Lips together teeth apart, never from this rule depart,' is easily said but difficult to practise if a clenching or grinding habit has been established. Placing a cotton pellet between the teeth with the advice, 'do not flatten it,' can be a reminder to keep the teeth apart but this, too, can be clenched. There are few habits more damaging to teeth, muscles, joints and tissues supporting denture bases, and every effort should be made to help patients control and prevent clenching. Occlusal and articular balance is therefore of first importance after seating a partial denture in order to prevent cusp interferences which can promote these parafunctional habits.

Domiciliary service

For carrying out impressions, jaw registrations and occlusal adjustment procedures in the home or institution, the requirements are upright seating with head support for the patient and illumination for the dentist. A straight-back chair with cushion for head support against the wall can be adequate for lower impressions, jaw registrations and occlusal corrections, provided that the dentist is prepared to kneel before the patient. The two-chair method with pillow on knee can be helpful for upper impressions and for simple restorative and surgical procedures (Fig. 7.5). Illumination can be provided by a reading lamp or a head lamp powered by batteries. The kitchen, with water and heat supply is the room of choice. A portable motor can be invaluable for making denture adjustments and portable boxes are available for carrying most home care instruments (Fig. 7.6).

Management decisions

Many elderly patients are not convinced of the need for complete dentitions and a pair of opposing posterior teeth (or less than this number) on both sides of the arch can provide adequate function. Replacement of anterior teeth is essential for appearance, and can be provided by a relatively simple appliance. Function and appearance are of great importance to the very elderly. The

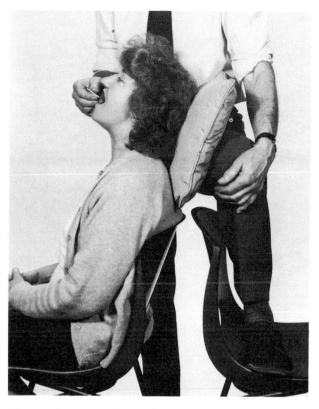

Fig 7.5   *The two chair method for head support.*

provision of comfortable teeth, both natural and artificial, is therefore a priority for them and a challenge to the dental profession. Where partial dentures are concerned, there is a wide range of choice in designs and materials but principles remain strict. These are: health, stability and comfort of existing teeth; the use of a surveyor for paths of insertion and retainer design; accuracy in occlusal registrations; and contingencies for further loss. Cost can be an insurmountable problem but where fees can be afforded the challenge to the dentist is all the greater. Brittleness of dentine and degeneration of pulps make the prognosis for abutment teeth uncertain. Decisions must be made with this knowledge in mind and with the cooperation of the patient. The design and choice of abutments is outside the scope of this text. Finally, hygiene of the remaining teeth, especially of the

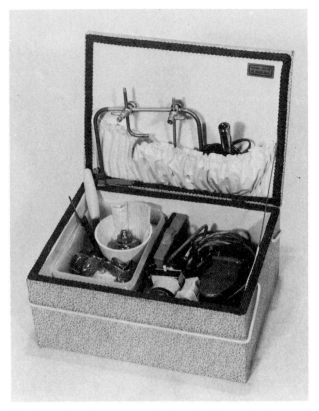

Fig 7.6   *The domiciliary box carrying facebow, headlamp, bowl, spatula, measured alginate, trays, spirit lamp, forceps for articulating paper, batteries for head-lamp, portable motor with foot switch.*

abutment teeth, by brush, tape, cotton bandage or woodstick cannot be too strongly emphasised.

OVERDENTURES

Before proceeding to the mangement of complete dentures on edentulous residual ridges, the advantages and disadvantages of overdentures for the elderly will be discussed. These dentures rest on two or more prepared root surfaces, usually rounded and not necessarily covered with metal, but the root canals will have been sterilised and filled. No attachment for the denture base will be advised or discussed in this text.

The loss of all teeth, particularly those in the mandible, is much feared by patients and dentists alike, and the reason lies in the failure of dentists to be certain of satisfying their patients' requirements and expectations in complete dentures. Some patients show a remarkable adaptability to the 'floating lower denture', but they are few in number and dentists should be thankful for them. Thus the retention of a few teeth, albeit root-filled and with crowns removed, gives to the patient a degree of security derived from proprioception through the periodontal membrane receptors and from the maintenance of the residual alveolar ridge around and between the abutment teeth.

There are four factors which should be evaluated and found favourable if teeth are to succeed as abutments for overdentures. These are: periodontal health; minimal caries activity; good root-filling prognosis; and favourable positions of the roots in the arch.

Periodontal health implies at least 6mm of healthy bone around the roots, minimal pockets, and a positive attitude by the patient to oral hygiene. Brushing the root surfaces is seldom enough and the towelling method previously mentioned can be effective if a one-inch bandage is folded and the folded edge inserted into the periodontal space. Patient cooperation for hygiene is therefore a necessity – and this is not always assured in the elderly.

Caries activity is not easily assessed and patients should be questioned on their early history of toothache and fillings, which can provide an indicator for the survival of overdenture abutments.

Root-filling prognosis should be based on a seal between canal and periodontal space, and the lamina dura around the apex should be intact. These teeth may have to bear the full load of masticatory function in addition to any clenching or grinding habits to which the patient may be subject which, of course, must be strongly discouraged from the start.

Abutment teeth should be carefully selected, with the two mandibular canines being optimal. Incisors and premolars are seldom successful but molars, especially if there is one on either side of the arch, can be effective. A recent contribution to the retention of overdentures is the use of magnets as suggested by Gillings (1984) Satisfactory magnetic retention has been produced by incorporating separate parts into the denture and on to the abutment tooth respectively. A useful text on the subject of overdentures is that of Brewer and Morrow (1975).

COMPLETE DENTURES

Requirements

Patients approach the loss of all teeth and the acceptance of complete dentures with attitudes that vary between the despair of premature ageing (however old they may be) and relief from prolonged suffering, and many with a combination of both. The responsibility of the dentist is greater than is perhaps realised. Improved appearance and comfortable eating are the chief expectations of the patient, and these must form the clinical requirements. An acceptable appearance is best provided at the time when the last incisor and canine teeth are to be removed and this will be the subject of the next two sections.

The function of comfortable eating requires posterior teeth with cusps that meet in balanced contact on closure in the empty mouth and are free from interfering contacts during lateral and protrusive gliding movements. When fulfilled, these requirements will allow patients to be unaware of their teeth when the mouth is empty and to use their teeth for shredding and chewing when food is eaten. If this can be performed on both sides simultaneously, mastication can often be fully restored to patients' satisfaction. Chopping the food may even become more efficient than chewing. The skill of providing balanced occlusion and free articulation, while retaining opposing cusps and fossae, is not easily achieved and cusps are often flattened in attempts to create balance. This will result in the food being squashed without penetration, so that mastication is impaired. In addition, balance in articular movements may then be difficult or even impossible to create, as when an increased incisor overlap has to be incorporated.

Balanced occlusion, free articulation and bilateral chewing will allow equal forces to be directed on both sides of the supporting residual ridges, with benefit to the stability of the dentures as well as to their retention. Reference to this requirement will be made in the section on occlusal adjustment.

The transition to complete dentures

The management of a prosthesis is made easier if the muscle activity required to support it is younger rather than older. The advice to have all remaining teeth removed and dentures placed earlier rather than later will not be accepted for this reason only, but it can help the patient to accept it where the loss of teeth seems to be inevitable. Further, this advice can be given to a 70-year-old patient, saying that it will be easier to manage the dentures at that time than five years later. This is especially true when the removal of teeth can be followed by the insertion of immediate dentures, where the artificial teeth can be placed in the position of their natural predecessors and where the dentures can be permanent. This principle can be made practicable by the operation of intraseptal alveolotomy, where space is created for the labial plate of the denture by removal of the septa between the extracted teeth.

Immediate dentures

Surgical procedures

The operation is best limited to the maxillary incisor and canine teeth and, when these are removed, triangular notches are cut at either end of the labial plate of bone, using side-cutting rongeur forceps. The interdental septa are then removed, using the same forceps, and the labial cortical plate of bone is collapsed against the lingual plate. Sutures are placed, thus permitting healing by first intention. Any postoperative swelling will provide a close fit between denture and tissue. New bone is subsequently deposited from the cortical plate inwards, and the denture remains closely fitting. This procedure has proved successful in my hands for 30 years and one 84-year-old patient lived to be 93, still wearing the immediate denture placed at the time of operation. Age, therefore, need not be a bar to such operative procedures.

The operation is not indicated in the mandibular arch, where both labial and lingual plates are of thicker bone and would not fracture in the same manner as in the maxillary bone. However, the residual bone can be smoothed by end-cutting rongeur forceps and this may allow the gum flaps to be sutured over the bone. The labial extension of the denture base should be kept as short as possible and should certainly not extend into the mucosa of the sulcus, otherwise there will be bruising. Subsequent additions can be made in acrylic resin after wound healing is complete. Thus the muscles of the lips and tongue, acting in` established patterns, will tend to stabilise the artificial teeth because they are in the same position as the natural teeth preceding them and age does not alter these patterns.

Setting the teeth

When the casts from the final impressions have been mounted, having used a facebow to transfer the maxillary cast and a pre-contact record on the retruded arc to mount the mandibular cast, the technician sets the posterior teeth; the jaw relations are then checked in the mouth. When returned to the laboratory for finishing, the canine, lateral and central incisors are removed, replacing each in succession with its artificial counterpart. It is important to seat the canine accurately before removing the plaster lateral, and similarly with the central. These are waxed to the palatal trial base and the procedures repeated for the other side. The trial denture is now removed and, from the area above these teeth, the dentist cuts away plaster to correspond with the additional space to be created by the surgical procedure described above. This should ensure that the labial flange of the denture has the same outline as the tissue it is replacing, thus preserving an unaltered appearance of the upper lip. Once cured, the dentures are returned to their mounting casts for refinements of occlusion. Following surgery they are seated and advice is given not to remove them for 48 hours. They can then be adjusted and, if necessary, remounted for occlusal corrections (see p. 199).

Dentists and patients alike may be apprehensive about so much surgery for an elderly person and it should not be undertaken lightly. Local anaesthesia, preferably incorporating an infra-orbital block and, with the physician's cooperation, some pre-medication, makes this a successful operation. If general anaesthesia is requested, the patient's physician should be consulted and an anaesthetist engaged. Admission to hospital should be considered. Recovery is almost always complete, with some swelling and haematoma as occasional after-effects. The denture is permanent but can be rebased in the area of the healed wound. A duplicate of this denture can be made (Thomson 1967) if required. A second permanent denture can, of course, be made but is not advised in view of the difficulties in restoring the correct tooth positions.

Unsatisfactory dentures

The consultation

This is the commonest problem expressed by elderly patients consulting a new dentist, and it can be difficult to discover the cause. A consultation away from the dental chair is advised, using a planned series of questions, but first the patient should be allowed to describe the problem in his own words. Salient points are noted. The objective then is to estimate whether the cause of trouble is one of support (condition of the denture-bearing tissues), retention (fit of the denture bases), stability (fit of the dentures during various functions required), or appearance: there may be more than one problem.

The questionnaire should not be too long, and the questions phrased in a kindly manner. Watching the patient's mouth in order to estimate the closest speaking space can give an indication of the occlusal vertical dimension (OVD); this is best seen with the 's' sounds. Ask the patient about eating, and whether one side is preferred. Where are the sore places and when do they occur? Do you clench or grind your teeth and when does this happen? Do you keep your dentures in overnight? Is the appearance different from your own teeth and do you have any smiling photographs before they were removed? Are there any other problems?

As mentioned in Chapter 5, an accompanying spouse or friend can act as an intermediary at the time and subsequently, but there are dangers of the second person dominating the patient.

The examination

Here the objectives are to confirm faults in retention, stability (mostly by occlusal errors and tooth positions), appearance and support. Before removing the dentures, an assessment is made of the appearance while smiling and speaking. It is necessary to look for any displacement of either denture, and any unfavourable forces being exerted by the tongue, lips or cheeks on the denture surfaces when the patient's mouth is wide open. Marks are then selected or made on the nose and chin, and the distance between them measured with the mandible in intercuspal position. This establishes the OVD. The patient is then asked to relax the mandible in order to adopt the rest position, so that the rest vertical dimension (RVD) can be measured. This should be 3mm below the OVD.

The dentures are then secured, either by fixative or by gentle holding with the forefinger and thumb of the left hand. The mandible is coaxed by the right hand into retruded closure, and any interference to bilateral contact noted. The mandibular denture is then removed and the RVD measured again. The RVD may now be found to be reduced, indicating that the tongue has made contact with the palate of the maxillary denture and caused the mandible to rise. The RVD may be further reduced after removal of the maxillary denture if the tongue makes contact with the palate. The border of the mandibular denture is assessed for contact with displaceable mucosa, and for over- or underextension. This assessment is then repeated for the maxillary denture. The residual ridges of both mandible and maxilla are then examined for causes of soreness and problems of support. Intra-oral radiographs may be helpful in discovering or confirming such causes.

Treatment plan

Many patients will request new dentures when considerations of treatment are discussed, especially if they think they are consulting a denture expert, and this can be difficult to resist. On the other hand, there are few faulty dentures that cannot be improved by adjustments to borders, to occlusion, and to the labial, buccal or lingual surfaces of the teeth and of the artificial mucosa.

Improvement procedures

Retention can normally be improved by adding to the borders of the denture bases, without altering the fitting (supporting) surfaces. If no alteration to the occlusal vertical dimension is planned, this can be more helpful as a preliminary measure than rebasing the whole denture surface. The border areas most likely to benefit from these additions are extensions to the 'vibrating line' in the maxillary denture and, in the mandibular denture, additions for improved seal in the anterior lingual, posterior lingual (determined by the mylohyoid muscles), and retro-molar pad regions. Materials for making these additions can be tracing stick compound (later to be replaced with processed acrylic resin) or a fast-setting acrylic resin with plasticiser, as a temporary measure.

Support for the dentures can often be improved by the surgical removal of sharp bone surfaces, such as mylohyoid ridges, enlarged mentalis tubercles and areas of bone giving rise to undercuts, often seen in the maxillary tuberosity regions. These procedures are best carried out by an oral surgeon.

Appearance can be improved by reference to pre-extraction photographs, to a radiographic assessment of the skeletal relations between mandible and maxilla (Thomson 1981), and to any problems of lip posture with the existing dentures. It may be necessary to remove and re-set the incisor teeth, but improvements can often be made by thinning or shortening the teeth. If it is decided to rebase dentures, alteration of tooth positions can be made at that time.

Stability is likely to benefit from:

1. Occlusal adjustment
2. Reshaping the muscle (polished) surfaces
3. Alteration of tooth positions
4. Rebasing the dentures
5. Rebasing with a soft lining
6. Eliminating sore places

1. Occlusal adjustment. This is defined as removal of selected areas of the teeth in order to restore intercuspal occlusion on the retruded horizontal and correct vertical position of the mandible, and to provide balanced articulation in lateral and protrusive contact movements.

Most texts on prosthodontics include procedures on occlusal adjustment and the following aspects are emphasised:

a. A face bow transfer of the maxillary denture to an adjustable articulator is made. This ensures that the maxillary denture will rotate on the same axis of opening and closure as the mandible does on its retruded axis.

b. A jaw relation record is made between the mandibular and maxillary teeth just prior to contact on the retruded axis of the mandible, thus allowing the same axis of opening and closing to be followed on the articulator as in the mouth. The angle of condyle descent is adjusted by a transferred protruded record, thus allowing the upper member of the articulator to copy the protruded movement of the mandible. The lateral movements are assumed to take place at the same angle.

c. These records are then used for mounting casts made for the dentures.

d. Equal contacts are developed, where necessary, between cusps and fossae on all posterior teeth, by deepening the fossae rather than flattening the cusps. This is achieved by trimming the **m**esial aspects of the maxillary (**u**pper) cusps or the **d**istal aspects of the mandibular (**l**ower) cusps. Hence MU DL. This provides for a more retruded position of the mandible on closure.

e. Freedom from interfering contacts in protrusive and working lateral movements is provided by trimming the **b**uccal **u**pper or **l**ingual **l**ower aspects of cusp ridges for working side and protrusive interference (BU LL). For non-working sides (the more damaging balancing interferences), the **m**esial-facing **i**nner aspects of the **b**uccal **l**ower cusps, or the **d**istal-facing **i**nner aspects of the **l**ingual **u**pper cusps, are trimmed (MI BL or DI LU).

It is always more effective to perform occlusal adjustments on an articulator using these transfer records and they can be inaccurate if a plain hinge instrument is used. Correct paths of movement between mouth and adjustable articulator will result in accurate contacts and valid adjustments. The question then arises: Why not use the mouth as an articulator? If the bases are securely sealed (by fixative if necessary), and a retruded path of closure can be made by the patient while the dentist (or, preferably, the dental nurse) holds the forceps (Pascal) carrying thin articulating paper, an accurate record of interfering contacts may be registered. If the dentist is sure of his objective and method, this procedure can prove successful.

When giving **domiciliary service**, face bow and jaw registrations can be made with the patient seated in a chair with the head supported by a cushion on the wall. The dentures will then have to be taken to the dental laboratory for mounting and adjustment. Alternatively, articulating paper records can be made, as described above, and the adjustments made in the home if a portable motor is available. Without a nurse to hold the forceps, practice is required to ensure seating of the dentures with the articulating paper in position.

2. Reshaping the muscle (polished) surfaces. Most dentures are finished so that the polished buccal and labial gum surfaces correspond in outline to those in the natural dentition. This can provide a good appearance, especially if the acrylic resin has a stippled finish. However, in elderly patients whose muscle activities have deteriorated, these surfaces may act as levers for displacement. Hollows may then be helpful for stability to engage: (a) the orbicularis oris muscles above and below the lips; (b) the 'modiolus effect' (Fish 1948) opposite the mandibular canines and premolars; (c) the triangularis muscles acting opposite the maxillary premolars; and (d) the buccinators acting horizontally above and below the necks of the maxillary and mandibular posterior teeth. Lee (1954) suggested ledges to engage the upper fibres of these muscles. The multi-muscled tongue normally lies with its greatest lateral convexity above the mandibular teeth and provides the lingual wall of the neutral zone, with the buccinators providing the buccal wall. The tip of the tongue normally lies on the lingual surfaces of the mandibular incisors, and a definite hollow here will encourage the tongue to rest on it. This can be of benefit to the stability of the denture, but the patient should be made aware of it and advised to 'keep touching the hollow when eating'. Finally, room for tongue activity can be created by removing and polishing areas on the palate, particularly above the lingual borders of the teeth.

3. Alteration of tooth positions. Unless otherwise advised, technicians will set up in Class I tooth relations, and there are occasions when this will be in conflict with the musculature of a Class II or III jaw relation. It is the dentist's responsibility to make an assessment of the jaw relation by lateral skull radiograph if need be, when the SNA–SNB angle can be measured (Thomson 1981). This will indicate the skeletal jaw relation: unless the tooth positions conform to this relation, the muscle activity will not tolerate the denture. Sometimes a short upper lip, a retruded or protruded chin, or an estimate by eye of the angle of the mandible will give an indication of the jaw reaction. Here again a smiling photograph, with the natural teeth still present, can prove helpful. Alteration of the incisor tooth positions to conform to the correct jaw relation (the teeth in the neutral zone) can result in a marked improvement in denture stability.

4. Rebasing the dentures. This procedure will solve nothing if the supporting surfaces of the dentures are filled with an impression material and the patient asked to close the teeth. The jaw relation will have been altered and the consequent occlusion will not be level. This will have a damaging effect on the stability and retention of the dentures. The following procedure is, therefore, suggested:

a. A record of the OVD is made with the existing dentures in place. This is measured by dividers on marks above and below the mouth. Any decision to increase or reduce the OVD is now made.

b. The impressions are made after ensuring that the existing bases are extended to displaceable mucosa by using tracing stick compound or other plastic material so that the final 'wash' impression covers these extensions but is not displaced by the supporting mucosa.

c. The dentures with these impressions are returned to the mouth and the occlusal position on the retruded axis is measured, using the same marks as previously. This is likely to be increased by 3–4mm from the original OVD due to the thickness of the wash impressions, especially if both dentures are being rebased. They are also likely to bear a tilted relation to each other. It is therefore necessary to make a face bow record of the position of the maxillary denture in relation to the arbitrary retruded axis, and a pre-contact jaw registration on this axis. Preference is given to the upright posture of the patient when making this registration.

d. The master casts are accurately notched on their bases so that they can be returned to their mounting casts after curing. The casts with the dentures are then mounted, using the records made. The dentures are taken from their casts and the impression material removed. Careful cleaning follows and the palate is cut out. The rest of the maxillary denture is then waxed to its cast at the position closest to its original seating. The mandibular denture is then placed against the maxillary denture at intercuspal occlusion and secured to it. The OVD is selected on the incisal guidance pin, the screw secured and the figure noted. The mandibular denture is then waxed to its master cast on the articulator.

e. The dentures with their casts are now removed from the mounting casts on the articulator, and the supporting surfaces are cured. They are then returned to the articulator, where the occlusion is checked and, if necessary, corrected.

This procedure is given in some detail because many rebased dentures fail when corrections for altered occlusion are not made. The dentist may think he has observed closure into previously established intercuspal positions when the impressions are made, but errors are almost certain if this is done while the impression is setting. The procedure also requires the services of a technician who understands the problems of copying paths of closure to and from occlusal positions and the advantages and limitations of adjustable articulators.

5. Rebasing with soft lining. When patients come with their dentures lined with cotton wool, something is wrong. Well-fitting acrylic resin bases can cause bruising to mucosa supported by sharp residual ridges, in spite of balanced occlusion and free articulation. A softer base material may therefore be indicated if surgery is not. Patients also buy soft lining materials and these can provide temporary relief, but the consequential alterations in the occlusion seldom give permanent comfort.

Existing soft lining materials may be classified as silicone elastomers and soft acrylics. Soft acrylic consists of a polymer powder (usually polyethyl methacrylate) and a monomer liquid with a phthalate plasticiser. While such materials have good adhesion to hard methacrylate, they tend to have poor elastic properties and harden rapidly because the plasticiser leaches out. Silicone soft liners polymerise at room temperature and have good elastic properties, but adhesion to the methacrylate is poor. They also tend to deteriorate in the mouth, and support the growth of *Candida albicans*. What is required, therefore, is to confer good adhesion on silicone polymers or to make a soft acrylic with a non-leachable plasticiser.

A commercially-available branched silicone polymer with a methacrylate group is a good compromise; it reacts with the methyl methacrylate polymer and adheres to it. Work has been done on polymerisable plasticisers, and a powdered elastomer with a higher methacrylate ester has been developed. This obviates the need for an external plasticiser and has responded favourably to peeling, shearing and tearing tests.

It has to be acknowledged that soft linings are not as soft as some patients would like, nor as well retained as some expect. They are also too thick for maxillary bases and they tend to harbour food debris but they have proved a comfort to some elderly mouths. The procedure is as for rebasing the denture, except that enough space must be left for a layer of new methyl methacrylate in order to provide the necessary adhesion between the two materials, as the soft lining will not adhere to processed acrylic resin.

6. Eliminating sore places. In spite of all the care that may have gone into making or improving dentures, sore places do occur. They may be caused not by occlusal faults but by overextensions in the impressions or by processing errors. If the residual ridges have mucosal folds which are duplicated on the cast, sharp edges will occur on the processed denture. There are few bases so stable that such edges will remain firmly in their corresponding folds during function. This is particularly true in mandibular bases where there is always some degree of movement, and these edges and ridges should be removed accurately and minimally. A well-tried procedure is as follows: the bruised area is dried and touched with pressure-indicating paste for which a good formula is equal parts of vaseline, powdered starch and zinc oxide. This is applied on the end of a sable paint brush; the area is kept dry while the dried denture is gently seated; the paste will transfer to the base, which can then be adjusted.

There are limitations to what can be done to improve a patient's unsatisfactory dentures, but improvements are always possible where there are diagnosable complaints. For the elderly patient confined to house or institution much can be done, but this depends on the planning and time available. Figure 7.6 illustrates a box which can carry an adequate prosthodontic kit. The attitude and circumstances of the patient may determine what is possible. Elderly patients, tired of adjustments to unsatisfactory dentures, often want to be rid of them and to begin again. These are the difficult problems and will be the topic of the next section.

New complete dentures

Before the first impression

When both patient and dentist are convinced that new dentures are the only solution to their common problem, warning should be given that the dentures will be like 'new shoes' and will require a period of adjustment. The patient should also be told that the tissues in general are shrinking, and the bone under the gum tissue is changing shape (resorbing), and that this will be accentuated if the patient clenches, grinds and presses on the teeth either while chewing or when the mouth is empty, and particularly the latter. Faults in previous dentures have to be assessed and corrected, because neither patient nor dentist wants to finish with similar or new problems. Confidence in one's technique is seldom enough to solve these problems in the elderly patient and not only should the dentist be certain of the principles involved in previous faults, and be able to correct them, but patients should be made aware that there are real problems in their mouths, and cautioned not to be over-optimistic. Flat or flabby ridges (support problems) should be demonstrated, habits should be explained, smiling photographs with natural teeth produced, wrinkles explained, and radiographs made of both residual ridges (three intra-oral maxillary and three mandibular should be adequate) for signs of retained roots, residual infection or uneven ridges. Notes should be made of rest vertical dimension and of size, colour and number of teeth to be used. It is not always necessary to supply 28 teeth: many patients have managed with many less in their natural dentitions, so why, suddenly, should there be 28 teeth taking up space where the tongue had previously been free to move?

Consideration should therefore be given to omitting the first molars or the second maxillary molars (which makes protrusive balance more easily achieved). As a result, the tongue will be given more freedom and greater ability to extend on top of the denture, thus aiding its stability. The patient should be advised of any reduction in the number of teeth and given an explanation. The unused teeth can be given to the patient in a sachet, with the assurance that they can be added to the denture if the need should arise.

Procedures

1. Impression making. The principles of maximal coverage of firm mucosa and extension to displaceable mucosa are advocated, taking account of functional anatomy. Old patients respond well to appeals for cooperation and will pull out their lower or upper lip when the loaded tray is being inserted. This attitude may help when it comes to the more difficult procedures of registering jaw relations. The dental nurse can be of help, too, in supporting the mandible or wiping the brow if the patient is in any distress. Impression materials should be fast-setting, and using them requires quick movements which should be rehearsed. Retching is no more common than in younger patients: topical or local anaesthesia can be provided for the soft palate if there is a problem.

2. Jaw registrations. There will always be differences of opinion on where to register the mandibular position. The view expressed here is that, as the retruded relation of mandible to maxilla and the arc of closing when retruded are reproducible, they should be used when transferring bases to the articulator. It is true that the elderly patient may not want to make the effort to pull the jaw back each time a swallow is made but the intercuspal occlusion so reached will provide a reassuring and stabilising position of closure. A facebow transfer of the maxillary base and a pre-contact registration of the mandibular base on the retruded axis will ensure that the arc of closure of the upper base on the articulator will correspond to the retruded arc of mandibular closure in the mouth. The operator must then make sure that the vertical component of occlusion is established at a level of 3mm above that of rest position. It can be helpful to check the mounting on the articulator before proceeding to set up the teeth, and this may be done by the split-cast or opposing pins method (Thomson 1981).

3. Correct tooth positions and muscle surfaces. Objectives for these features have already been stated (p. 201) but they are even less easily achieved when making new dentures. The following procedure may prove helpful: after mounting the bases, compound rims are added, softened and inserted; the patient is asked to purse the lips and swallow vigorously; the bases and rims are removed and the excess compound is trimmed until

they appproximate the outlines of the tooth and gingival surfaces; an adhesive is now applied followed by a thin mix of
alginate; the bases and rims are re-inserted and the patient is
asked to purse the lips gently, whereupon an indication of tooth
position and gum outline may be deduced (L'Estrange 1974).

4. Occlusion and articulation. Emphasis has already been
given to the need for cusps in order to provide good occlusal
function (p. 194). However, free articulation for these cusps
should not be introduced at the expense of vertical incisor overlap where this is required in order to provide correct tooth
positions. The skill of providing balanced articulation belongs to
the technician but the dentist is well advised to learn the rules and
how to apply them. After completion, the dentures should be
worn for two days and then remounted using a pre-contact
registration. Occlusal adjustment may then be necessary (see
p. 199).

5. Advice on the use of dentures. It is perhaps late in the day to
advise elderly patients on how to eat but a few imperative phrases
may help:

> Place the food under the tongue and let it get wet with
> saliva.
> Divide it into two lots and load both sides.
> Eat on both sides at the same time.
> Chop rather than chew on the back teeth.
> Avoid letting the teeth touch while eating.
> Close on the teeth only to swallow the near liquid bolus.
> When not eating keep the teeth apart.
> Keep the tip of the tongue touching the backs of the lower
> front teeth at all possible times and especially when eating.
> Use the cheeks and sides of the tongue to keep the food
> loaded on to the back teeth.
> Remove the dentures overnight and keep in a cleansing
> solution (see p. 189).

Obviously, one does not reel off all these instructions in succession but, as a good general dictum, patients can be told to
chew with the back teeth and on both sides at once, with the
tongue kept forward.

There are patients in whose mouths much resorption has taken place and both mentalis tubercles and mylohyoid ridges are not only sharp but the muscles attached to them are above the level of the residual ridges. This makes the stable and comfortable seating of a denture during function almost impossible. Some patients have learned to manage such dentures and they do perform miracles with tongue, lips and cheeks but for the most part such mouths are a heartbreak to dentist and patient alike. Surgery to remove these ridges and tubercles and to cut back the muscle attachments involved has improved the support for many such patients, but it is not easy to persuade anyone in his late seventies to have more surgery in a mouth where much suffering has already been experienced. There is no point in saying that this situation might have been prevented by complete dentures or pre-prosthetic surgery at an earlier age.

DENTAL IMPLANTS

The need for something more than good intentions to solve the problems of missing teeth has stimulated the development of highly sophisticated dental implants. There is nothing new in the idea of replacing lost teeth by transplantation or implantation; there are reports covering a variety of materials used in past centuries, including human and animal teeth, plant materials and different metals. Significant in the descriptions of all these authors is the absence of any claim of prolonged success. Even today, despite the availability of new materials and the exercise of much technical ingenuity, the dominant theme in the literature on dental implants is the uncertainty of success.

The principles followed in constructing different types of dental implants, and the range of materials in use, have been comprehensively described by Johns (1976). Compatibility of the implant material is obviously essential and, in the search for an ideal material, metals, polymers, ceramics and vitreous carbon have all been put to the test. Cobalt chromium, available in most dental laboratories, has good biocompatibility but low strength and poor ductility. In 1969 Branemark et al. reported their early studies on the long-term stability of intra-osseous titanium implants, and all current aspects of dental implants using this metal are covered in the published Proceedings (1983) of a conference on osseointegration held in Toronto. The method advocated for constructing the titanium fixtures is not, however, for the tyro. It entails a two-part design, the first of which is fitted intraosseously and remains buried for a lengthy period of inactivity until integrated into the bone structure; the occlusal superstructure is added subsequently. This may be too much to ask of an elderly patient in terms of time and cost, and is better suited to younger subjects. A helpful survey of current implant research is that of Hobkirk (1983).

REFERENCES

Branemark P.-I., Breine U., Adell R., Hansson B. O., Lindstrom J., Ohlsson A. (1969). Intra-osseous anchorage of dental prostheses. Scand. J. Plast. Reconstr. Surg.; **3**: 81–100.

Brewer A. A., Morrow R. M. (1980). *Overdentures*. St Louis: The C. V. Mosby Company.

Craddock F. W. (1956). *Prosthetic Dentistry*, 3rd edn. pp. 320–2. London: Kimpton.

Fish E. W. (1948). *Principles of Full Denture Prosthesis*. 4th edn. pp. 36–7. London: Staples Press.

Gillings B. R. D. (1984). Magnetic denture retention system: inexpensive and efficient. *Int. Dent. J.*; **34**: 184–97.

Hobkirk J. A. (1983). Progress in implant research. *Int. Dent. J.*; **33**: 341–9.

Jacobson T. E., Krol A. J. (1982). Rotational path removable partial denture designs. *J. Prosthet. Dent.*; **48**: 370–6.

Johns R. B. (1976). Dental implants. In *Scientific Foundations of Dentistry* (Cohen B., Kramer I. R. H., eds.) pp. 663–9. London: William Heinemann Medical Books.

Lee J. H. (1954). The form of the denture surfaces. *Dent. Rec.*; **74**: 318–20.

L'Estrange P. R., Pullen-Warner E. (1969). Sectional dentures, a simplified method of attachment. *Dent. Practit.*; **19**: 379–81.

L'Estrange P. R. (1974). *Variation in human oral function with alteration in morphology*. Ph.D. thesis. University of London.

Proceedings of the 1982 Toronto Conference on Osseointegration in Clinical Dentistry. Reprinted from the J. Prosthet. Dent. Vol. **49**, No. 6 (June 1983) and Vol. **50**, Nos. 1, 2 and 3 (July, August, September, 1983). St Louis: The C. V. Mosby Company.

Thomson H. (1967). Duplication of complete dentures. *Dent. Practit.*; **17**: 173–5.

Thomson H. (1981). *Occlusion in Clinical Practice*, pp. 5–6, 126–8. Bristol: Wright PSG.

Index